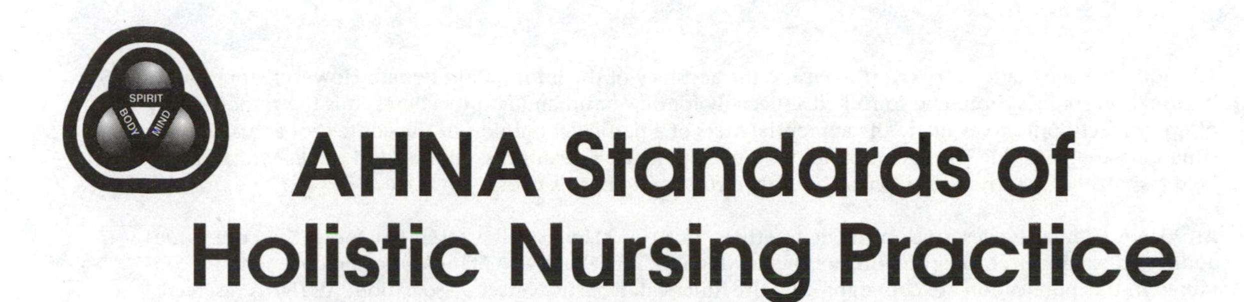

AHNA Standards of Holistic Nursing Practice

Guidelines for Caring and Healing

Noreen Cavan Frisch, PhD, RN, HNC, FAAN
Chair and Professor
Department of Nursing
Cleveland State University
Cleveland, Ohio

Barbara Montgomery Dossey, MS, RN, HNC, FAAN
Director
Holistic Nursing Consultants
Santa Fe, New Mexico

Cathie E. Guzzetta, PhD, RN, HNC, FAAN
Nursing Research Consultant
Children's Medical Center of Dallas and
Parkland Health & Hospital Systems
Director
Holistic Nursing Consultants
Dallas, Texas

Johanne A. Quinn, PhD, RN, HNC
Chair and Professor
Department of Nursing
King College
Bristol, Tennessee

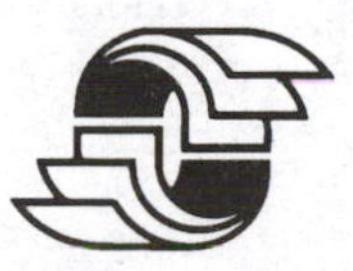

AN ASPEN PUBLICATION®
Aspen Publishers, Inc.
Gaithersburg, Maryland
2000

Library of Congress Cataloging-in-Publication Data

American Holistic Nurses' Association
AHNA standards of holistic nursing practice : guidelines for caring and healing /
Noreen Frisch . . . [et al.].
p. ; cm.
Includes bibliographical references and index.
ISBN 0-8342-1045-2
1. Holistic nursing—Standards. 2. Holistic nursing. I. Title: Standards of holistic nursing practice. II. Title: Holistic nursing practice. III. Frisch, Noreen Cavan. IV. Title.
[DNLM: 1. Holistic Nursing—Standards—United States. WY 86.5 A512a 2000]
RT42.A425 2000
610.73′02′1873—dc21 00-025297

Editorial Services: Ruth Bloom
Library of Congress Catalog Card Number: 00-025297
ISBN: 0-8342-1045-2

Printed in the United States of America

1 2 3 4 5

This book is dedicated to
all Holistic Nurses
and to the American Holistic Nurses' Association
"The Mission of the AHNA Is To Unite Nurses in Healing"

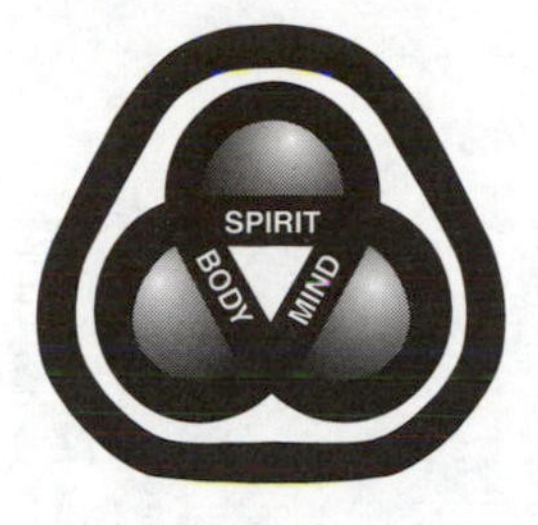

CONTENTS

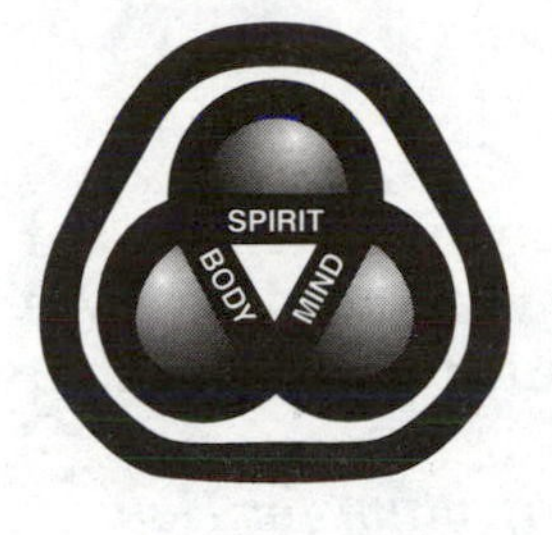

PREFACE

The first vision of this book came to us in the early 1990s when we were making initial attempts to identify the skills and competencies that were demonstrated by holistic nurses in the United States. Questions such as "Is there really a specialty within nursing called *holistic nursing*?" and "What defines the *holistic nurse* as compared to others who practice nursing?" led us to embark on a process that has lasted nearly a decade. We worked with many in the American Holistic Nurses' Association (AHNA) to define and describe the practice of holistic nursing. We published a description of holistic nursing in addition to position papers on social issues and on the support of a healthful environment. We drafted and approved a code of ethics for holistic nurses. And, finally, we began a process to publish standards of holistic nursing practice.

The process leading to this work is well described by Barbara Dossey, MS, RN, HNC, FAAN in the introduction to this book. We worked through three major revisions of these standards to come to the version presented here. While we know that standards of practice are continually evolving, we present the reader with Standards of Holistic Nursing Practice that are based on consensus of many within the field who are striving to keep the practice of nursing at its highest level—a practice that identifies every person as whole and attempts to meet the needs and expectations of each client of nursing. We see the nurse as a holistic being able to form a positive therapeutic relationship with a client. We see nursing as caring and healing. We see nursing as being grounded in science and art, composed equally of logic and intuition. We see nursing as guided by research and directed by compassion. We present this work to assist nurses to develop wholly and to become prepared for certification as holistic nurses.

This book is organized to follow the Standards of Holistic Nursing Practice, 3rd Revision, adopted by AHNA in 2000. There are five Core Values, which provide a framework for practice: Holistic Philosophy and Education; Holistic Ethics, Theories, and Research; Holistic Nurse Self-Care; Holistic Communication, Therapeutic Environment, and Cultural Diversity; and the Holistic Caring Process. Each of these five Core Values is presented as a chapter in this book. We have presented the accepted wording for each Standard of Practice, and defined and described the major concepts inherent in each Standard. We have suggested nursing activities that demonstrate compliance with the Standards. Lastly, through the use of Case Studies, we have prepared examples of nurses in practice who are either meeting or not meeting the Standards. We hope to illustrate to all the many challenges involved in nursing practice that is truly holistic.

This book is to be used as a companion to the *Core Curriculum for Holistic Nursing* (1997), edited by Barbara Dossey. The *Core Curriculum* draws heavily on the Standards of Practice and delineates the knowledge base for holistic nursing. The *Core Curriculum* provides a guide for applying the knowledge to holistic practice to meet nursing's holistic ideals.

Following the introduction, Core Values 1 through 4 define and illustrate the philosophy, the commitment to education, the ethics, and the incorporation of theory, research, and communication skills to practice. Further, these first four Core Values include acknowledgment of the need to provide culturally sensitive care and present the expectation and need that every holistic nurse engage in self-care. The fifth Core Value—the Holistic Caring Process—is perhaps of greatest importance, as it is the culmination of the other four with the knowledge base detailed in the *Core Curriculum*. As such, Core Value 5, while following the same format as the work presented in the other four Core Values, is presented in great detail to set out a guide for all nursing care.

The Appendixes of this book present additional resources that we believe will be useful to our readership. Appendix A is a Self-Assessment Tool for nurses to use in evaluating their own progress in incorporating these Standards into their practice on a day-to-day basis. Appendix B presents AHNA's Holistic Nursing Core Values Audit. Appendix C lists certificate programs that are endorsed by AHNA. Appendix D is a list of graduate nursing programs in the United States that offer a specialty in holistic nursing. Appendix E provides an example of how to incorporate the Standards with a holistic modality.

As first author and editor of this book, I wish to thank my co-authors and friends, Cathie Guzzetta, PhD, RN, HNC, FAAN and Johanne Quinn, PhD, RN, HNC, who very ably contributed their work and their expertise to the development of the Core Values. Further, I wish to particularly thank my dear friend and colleague, Barbara Dossey, with whom I have worked for over a decade to develop ideas, draft the first version of the Standards of Holistic Nursing Practice in 1993, complete a national survey to identify the elements of holistic nursing practice, and present this book to nurses who share our interest in holism. It is our hope that this book will assist our readers to reflect on nursing and to help bring holistic ideals back as we move forward in the 21st century.

Noreen Cavan Frisch, PhD, RN, HNC, FAAN

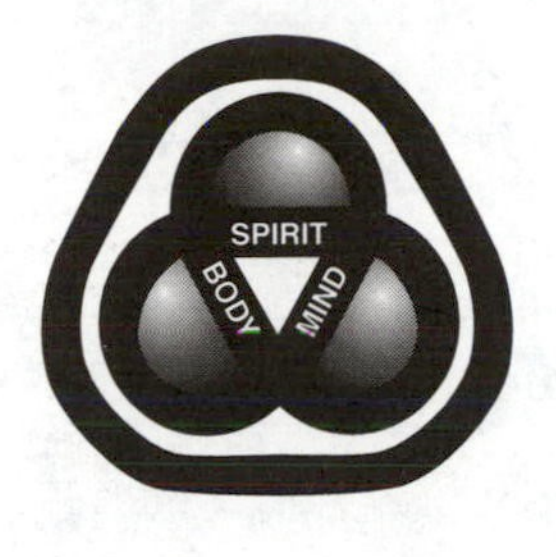

ACKNOWLEDGMENTS

The authors wish to gratefully acknowledge holistic nurses who, over years of practice, have defined a nursing specialty based on caring, compassion, holism, and wisdom. Together, we seek to achieve practice in keeping with these standards and worthy of the designation holistic nursing. We also acknowledge the fellowship of holistic nurses found in the American Holistic Nurses Association—the association that brought us together with many of the finest nurses in the world.

Special thanks are due to the staff of Aspen Publishers, who provided us with support, advice, and creativity during the process of developing this book. Those persons include ***Martha Sasser***, Editor Director, Patient Care; ***Mary Anne Langdon***, Senior Development Editor, who kept us on schedule; and the person who feels like a dear friend—***Ruth Bloom***, Managing Editor—Books, for attention to details and kind support.

Most of all, the four of us wish to thank those in our lives who believe in us and provide support and encouragement for projects that take on a life of their own and become our lives for an important period of time. These wonderful persons are: ***Larry and Mira Frisch, Larry Dossey, Phillip, Angela and Phillip C. Guzzetta,*** and ***John, Stephen, Beth, and Brian Quinn,*** and ***Lisa Johnston***—we thank them for their presence.

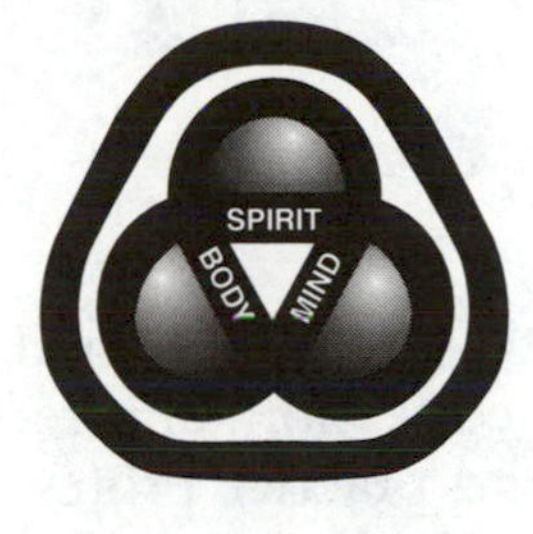

INTRODUCTION

Barbara Montgomery Dossey

From its inception in 1980, the American Holistic Nurses' Association (AHNA) has been the leader in the education of holistic principles, practices, and guidelines. The Association predicted that holistic principles, caring, healing, and the integration of complementary and alternative therapies would emerge into mainstream health care.

Holistic nursing is a philosophy and a model that integrates concepts of presence, healing, and holism. These concepts are based on broad and eclectic academic principles that incorporate a sensitive balance between art and science, analytic and intuitive skills, and the interconnectedness of body, mind, and spirit.

HISTORY AND DEVELOPMENT OF HOLISTIC NURSING

One of the driving forces behind the holistic nursing movement in the United States was the formation of AHNA. In 1980, founder Charlotte McGuire and 75 founding members began the national organization in Houston, Texas. AHNA has as its mission to unite nurses in healing with a focus on holistic principles of health, preventive education, and the integration of allopathic and complementary caring-healing modalities to facilitate care for the whole client and significant others. There are now many nurse clinicians, educators, authors, and researchers who are key figures in holistic nursing at university-based schools of nursing, professional practice environments, and nursing organizations outside of the AHNA.

The key published AHNA works are the *Journal of Holistic Nursing* (a quarterly journal published by Sage Publications, Inc.), *Beginnings* (AHNA monthly newsletter), *American Holistic Nurses' Association Core Curriculum for Holistic Nursing* (Aspen Publishers, Inc., 1997), *Holistic Nursing: A Handbook for Practice, Third Edition* (Aspen Publishers, Inc., 2000), and the *AHNA Standards of Holistic Nursing Practice* (Aspen Publishers, Inc., 2000).

ACKNOWLEDGMENTS: The AHNA would like to thank all committee members for their work and dedication to the 2000 revisions of the *AHNA Standards of Holistic Nursing Practice*.

AHNA ORGANIZATIONAL DEVELOPMENT PROCESS

The goals and endeavors of the AHNA have continued to map conceptual frameworks and the blueprint for holistic nursing practice, education, and research, which is the most complete way to conceptualize and practice professional nursing. Two major challenges have emerged in the 21st century. The first is to integrate the concepts of technology, mind, and spirit into nursing practice; the second is to further create and integrate models for health care that guide the healing of self and others.

To meet these two challenges, the AHNA undertook a five-year organizational development process from 1993 to 1998 that included the following five areas:

1. Identification of the steps toward national certification in 1993–1994;
2. Revision of the 1990 *AHNA Standards of Holistic Nursing Practice*, completed in 1995;
3. A role delineation study, the *Inventory of Professional Activities and Knowledge Statements of a Holistic Nurse* (IPAKHN), completed in 1997;
4. A national holistic nursing certification examination, completed in 1997; and
5. Major revisions of the 1995 *AHNA Standards of Holistic Nursing Practice*, completed in 1999 with additional editorial changes in January 2000.

This text, the *AHNA Standards of Holistic Nursing Practice*, is based on the AHNA developmental process and presents the latest revision of the Standards that is inherent in the continued development of holistic nursing. The following overview provides a historical perspective of the AHNA and its endeavors to assist holistic nurses, clinicians, educators, researchers, and students to meet today's challenges and to advance knowledge, practice, and research to further expand the processes of caring and healing.

CERTIFICATION IN HOLISTIC NURSING

In 1992, a four-phase AHNA Certificate Program in Holistic Nursing began. On completion of the program, a nurse was awarded a certificate in holistic nursing. In 1994, the AHNA Leadership Council appointed an AHNA Task Force Committee to explore the steps toward the development of holistic nursing certification through a national certification examination.

The AHNA Leadership Council appointed an AHNA Certification Committee to serve as the governing body to oversee the process of certification of holistic nurses by examination until a separate certification corporation was established. In 1997, the AHNA Certification Board established a separate 501C-6 organization, the American Holistic Nurses' Certification Corporation (AHNCC), to act as the credentialing arm of the AHNA to administer the AHNA Certification Examination. The AHNCC now has six directors who are voting members, and two non-voting members, one of whom is the President-elect of the AHNA Leadership Council. All of the Directors who serve on the AHNCC have been chosen for their skill in and knowledge of the process of certification. There is a public member who is not a nurse.

The AHNCC is an autonomous body with administrative independence in matters pertaining to certification. The AHNCC maintains a collaborative relationship with AHNA in order to set standards for the practice of holistic nursing. The AHNCC is not involved with the continuing education, endorsement, or accreditation activities of the AHNA. As the first step toward eligibility to take the national holistic nursing certification examination, a nurse must submit a qualitative assessment in the form of a portfolio for review by the AHNCC.

AHNCC Definition of Certification

The AHNCC defines certification as a qualifying process attesting that an individual, who is already practicing as a registered nurse and demonstrating basic nursing competencies, has met predetermined criteria for advanced or specialized practice. In relation to holistic nursing certification, the nurse must demonstrate competencies of specialized nursing practice encompassing holism.

The purpose of a certification process is to provide nurses with a standard they can be measured against, and to be able to declare to the community at large that certain individuals are competent to practice holistic nursing as defined by the *AHNA Standards of Holistic Nursing Practice.*

Development of Holistic Nursing Certification Examination

A major concern in the development and administration of a certification examination is determining adequate content validity. Content validity addresses the extent to which the test specifications reflect the knowledge and skills required of a holistic nurse. To ensure adequate content validity, a certification board must establish an appropriate table of specifications for use as a basis for test construction. This table of specifications, when analyzed, is called a *blueprint.* The blueprint needs to comprehensively detail the professional activities and knowledge areas that the examination should cover, as well as the number of items that should be written for each area. To accurately reflect holistic nursing practice, the AHNA Certification Examination must adhere to these professional activities and knowledge.

Documentation of Content Validity

To establish the content validity of the AHNA Certification Examination, a three-year role delineation study, Inventory of Professional Activities and Knowledge of a Holistic Nurse (IPAKHN Survey), was conducted between 1994 and 1997. The IPAKHN Survey analysis provided the content validity for the AHNCC certification examination.

Through practice analysis, sometimes called job analysis or role delineation, the content domain that will be measured by the certification examination is defined. This step in the test development process is essential for the validity of a certification examination. In the practice analysis study conducted by the AHNA, the activities and knowledge basic to current holistic nursing practice were determined through administration of a structured inventory to a representative sample of holistic nurses. This detailing of current practice then served as the basis for the development of test specifications for the AHNA Certification Examination.

Conducting the Role Delineation Study

This three-year endeavor was successfully completed by the dedicated work of three committees: the AHNA Task Force Committee, the Advisory Committee, and the Corresponding Committee. The 6-member AHNA Task Force Committee appointed the second committee, a 13-member Advisory Committee composed of the AHNA Leadership Council and select AHNA members, and the third committee, a 24-member Corresponding Committee composed of other recognized holistic nurse members and nonmembers. Members were selected carefully and systematically from holistic nursing experts to ensure a diversity of holistic nurse representation from practice, education, research, and administration.

AHNA STANDARDS OF HOLISTIC NURSING PRACTICE REVISIONS PROCESS

In late 1997, the AHNA Leadership Council gave the directive to the AHNA Standards of Practice Task Force Committee to further refine the 1995 *AHNA Standards of Holistic Nursing Practice*, which were divided into two parts and nine Core Values:

Part I: Discipline of Holistic Nursing Practice

Core Value 1. Holistic Philosophy
Core Value 2. Holistic Foundation
Core Value 3. Holistic Ethics
Core Value 4. Holistic Nursing Theories
Core Value 5. Holistic Nursing and Related Research
Core Value 6. Holistic Nursing Process

Part II: Caring and Healing of Clients and Significant Others

Core Value 7. Meaning and Wholeness
Core Value 8. Client Self-Care
Core Value 9. Health Promotion

Throughout 1998, an extensive five-step revision process of the *AHNA Standards of Holistic Nursing Practice* was achieved as follows:

Step 1: Literature Review, IPAKHN Survey Data Analysis, and Expert Reviews

The eight-member AHNA Standards of Practice Task Force Committee used as a foundation for the revision process the IPAKHN Survey data analysis recommendations. Since the IPAKHN Survey was created after an extensive literature review of the *Journal of Holistic Nursing* (1985–1995), *Holistic Nursing Practice* (1985–1995), and numerous other holistic nursing journals, holistic-related books, and research, the Task Force reviewed these same journals from 1996–1998 as well as *Essential Readings in Holistic Nursing* (1998) as a basis for the latest revisions.

In early 1998, the AHNA Standards of Practice Task Force Committee also announced the revision process in *Beginnings*, the newsletter of AHNA, thus involving the AHNA membership, those holistic nurses who had completed the qualitative assessment portfolio, and other recognized holistic nurse experts. Following this announcement, significant suggestions were submitted to the AHNA Task Force that were included in the first step of the revision process. Expert AHNA holistic nurses were invited to participate on one of the two committees, the Advisory Committee or the Review Committee.

Step 2: Review Process

Following Step 1, the AHNA Standards of Practice Task Force Committee incorporated the suggestions and additional data from the literature review and the IPAKHN Survey Analysis that reflected the most recent holistic nursing professional activities, knowledge, and caring-healing modalities. Based on this review and the additional comments, deletions, modifications, and recommendations by expert nurses, six areas were further refined and developed:

1. the AHNA holistic nursing description was expanded
2. guidelines were stated for better utilization and integration of the Standards in clinical practice, education, and research
3. interventions most frequently used in holistic nursing practice were identified based on the IPAKHN Survey data analysis
4. holistic nursing practice definitions were identified and described
5. a summary page of five Core Value statements was developed
6. the five Core Values were followed by Standards of Practice to reflect the dynamic art and science of holistic nursing practice.

Step 3: AHNA Standards of Practice Advisory Committee

Following Step 2, the revised AHNA Standards of Practice were next sent to the 24-member Advisory Committee, who gave additional comments, modifications, and recommendations. Step 3 involved five subsequent revision rounds by the AHNA Task Force Committee before consensus was achieved. It was again sent to the Advisory Committee for additional comments, modifications, and recommendations, which were incorporated.

Step 4: AHNA Standards of Practice Review Committee

Following Step 3, the revised AHNA Standards of Practice were next sent to the 24-member Review Committee, who gave additional comments, deletions, modifications, and recommendations. Step 4 involved three subsequent revision rounds by the AHNA Task Force Committee before consensus was achieved. It was again sent to the Review Committee for additional comments, deletions, modifications, and recommendations, which were incorporated.

The second phase of Step 4 involved a review by a 10-member AHNA Leadership Committee, who gave additional comments, deletions, modifications, and recommendations. Step 4 involved only one round by the AHNA Task Force Committee before consensus was achieved.

Following the revision process fourth round of responses from the AHNA Task Force Committee, the Advisory Committee, the Review Committee, and the Leadership Committee consensus on the revised *AHNA Standards of Holistic Nursing Practice* was achieved.

Step 5: AHNA Standards of Practice Leadership Council

Following Step 4, the final draft of the revised *AHNA Standards of Holistic Nursing Practice* was submitted to the AHNA Leadership Council prior to the June 1999 AHNA Board meeting. After a discussion of the revisions, a final vote of approval came to accept the revised *AHNA Standards of Holistic Nursing Practice*. These revisions were then presented at the annual AHNA Conference June 1999 AHNA Business Meeting in Scottsdale, Arizona. The revised AHNA Standards received a vote of approval by the AHNA membership. Minor editorial changes were approved by the AHNA Leadership Council in January 2000.

The *AHNA Standards of Holistic Nursing Practice* (see pp. xxiii–xxxv) now contains the following five Core Values (Figure I–1):

Core Value 1. Holistic Philosophy and Education
Core Value 2. Holistic Ethics, Theories, and Research
Core Value 3. Holistic Nurse Self-Care
Core Value 4. Holistic Communication, Therapeutic Environment, and Cultural Diversity
Core Value 5. Holistic Caring Process

CONCLUSION

The *AHNA Standards of Holistic Nursing Practice* provide a blueprint and guidelines for holistic practice, education, and research. These Standards guide clinicians, educators, researchers, nurse managers, and administrators in the professional activities, knowledge, and performance that are relevant to holistic nursing practice, education, research, and management. The identified Standards of Practice under each Core Value statement reflect a consensus of the necessary requirements to practice holistic nursing on a day-to-day basis. Specific professional activities can be linked to knowledge, practice, and research areas when planning undergraduate, graduate, and staff development curricula.

The *AHNA Standards of Holistic Nursing Practice* can serve as a guide when planning clinical conferences, clinical objectives, course requirements, and clinical and educational outcomes, and when writing test items so that all endeavors have more relevance to the actual practice of holistic nursing. They also provide an excellent basis for future research in areas of holistic nursing such as:

- Determining holistic guidelines and caring-healing modalities to help clients be in harmony with the changes that occur throughout the life span.
- Examining caring-healing modalities in nursing and health care practice that can facilitate healing, and determine which ones work, for which conditions, and with what results.

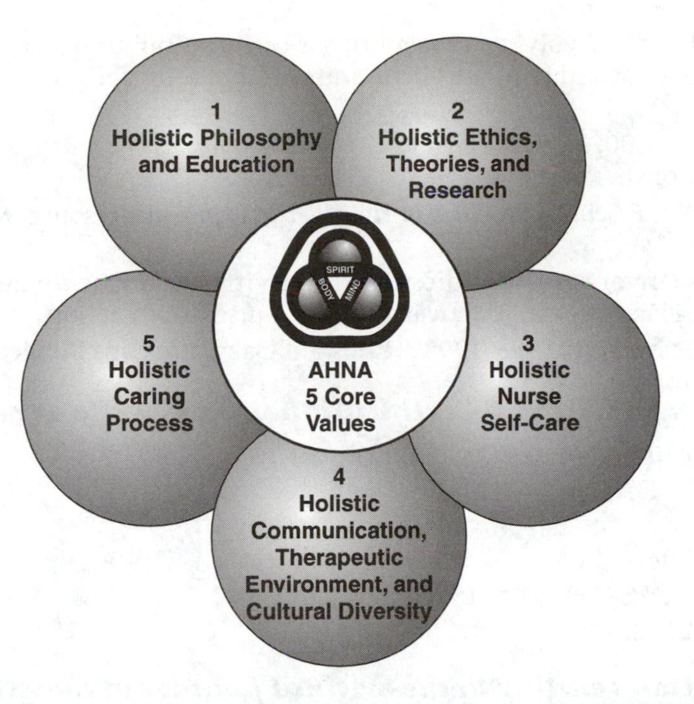

Figure I–1 The Five Core Values Embodied in the Standards of Holistic Nursing Practice of the American Holistic Nurses' Association (AHNA). *Source:* Copyright © American Holistic Nurses' Association (AHNA).

- Exploring the value that clients and their families attach to caring-healing modalities, and the value that nurses attach to them.
- Evaluating modes of integrating concepts of holistic nursing in curricula development, mission statements, inservice education, seminars, and research.
- Investigating anticipated or actual solutions or complications that result from holistic nursing and caring-healing interventions.
- Comparing the roles of newly certified holistic nurses with those nurses not certified, which could be accomplished through direct observation.
- Evaluating whether outcomes differ when clients interact with nurses who practice caring-healing modalities compared to interaction with nurses who do not use caring-healing modalities.

Holistic nurses can reduce the devastating effects of crisis and illness of individuals by using the *AHNA Standards of Holistic Nursing Practice* that incorporate bio-psycho-social-spiritual human dimensions and caring-healing modalities. These Standards serve as bridges for holistic nurses to understand more fully the emotions and meanings involved in clients' illness, crises, and life events. They also assist nurses in their own journey toward wholeness and healing.

RESOURCES

Dossey, B., ed. 1997. *American Holistic Nurses' Association Core Curriculum for Holistic Nursing*. Gaithersburg, MD: Aspen Publishers, Inc.

Dossey, B., et al. 1998. Evolving a blueprint for certification: Inventory of professional activities and knowledge of a holistic nurse. *Journal of Holistic Nursing* 16, no. 1: 33–56.

Dossey, B., et al. 2000. *Holistic Nursing: A Handbook for Practice,* 3rd ed. Gaithersburg, MD: Aspen Publishers, Inc.

Guzzetta, C. 1998. *Essential Readings in Holistic Nursing*. Gaithersburg, MD: Aspen Publishers, Inc.

IPAKHN Survey (Inventory of Professional Activities and Knowledge of a Holistic Nurse). 1997. Flagstaff, AZ: American Holistic Nurses' Association.

Journal of Holistic Nursing. 1996–1998. Thousand Oaks, CA: Sage Publications, Inc.

For details on the AHNCC Certification process write or call:

American Holistic Nurses' Association
2733 E. Lakin Drive
Suite 2
Flagstaff, AZ 86004
Phone: (800) 278-AHNA or (520) 526-2196
Fax: (520) 526-2752

For information relating to the original founder of holistic nursing:

Dossey, B. 2000. *Florence Nightingale: Mystic, Visionary, Healer*. Springhouse, PA: Springhouse Corporation.

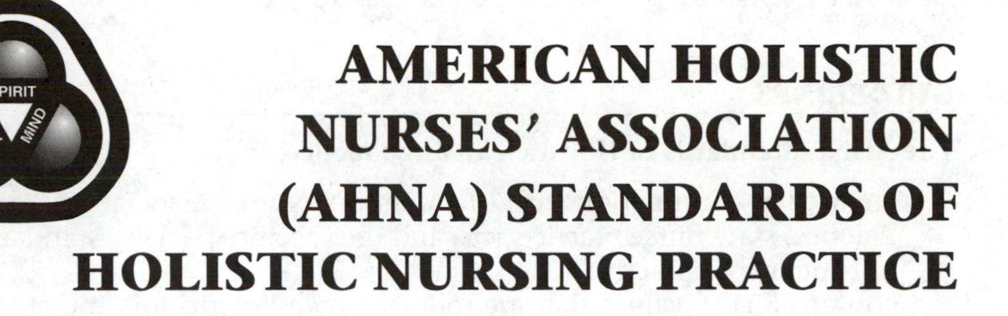

AMERICAN HOLISTIC NURSES' ASSOCIATION (AHNA) STANDARDS OF HOLISTIC NURSING PRACTICE

GUIDELINES

The AHNA Standards of Holistic Nursing Practice:

- are used in conjunction with the American Nurses Association Standards of Practice, state nurse practice acts, and the specific specialty standards where holistic nurses practice.
- contain 5 core values that are followed by a description and standards of practice action statements. Depending on the setting or area of practice, holistic nurses may or may not use all of these action statements.
- draw on modalities derived from a number of explanatory models, of which biomedicine is only one model.
- reflect the diverse nursing activities in which holistic nurses are engaged.
- serve holistic nurses in personal life, clinical and private practice, education, research, and community service.

AHNA HOLISTIC NURSING PRACTICE DEFINITIONS

Allopathic/Traditional Therapies: medical, surgical, invasive and noninvasive diagnostic treatments, procedures, including medications.

Caring-Healing Interventions: nontraditional therapies that can interface with traditional medical and surgical therapies; may be used as complements to conventional medical and surgical treatments; also called alternative/complementary/integrative therapies or interventions. See list of interventions most frequently used in holistic nursing practice.

Client of Holistic Nursing: an individual, family, group, or community of persons who is engaged in interactions with a holistic nurse in a manner respectful of each client's subjective experience about health, health beliefs, values, sexual orientation, and personal preferences.

Cultural Competence: the ability to deliver health care with knowledge of and sensitivity to cultural factors that influence the health behavior of the person.

Environment: everything that surrounds the person, both the external and the internal (physical, mental, emotional, and spiritual) environment as well as patterns not yet understood.

Healing: the process of bringing together aspects of oneself, body-mind-spirit, at deeper levels of inner knowing leading toward integration and balance with each aspect having equal importance and value; can lead to more complex levels of personal understanding and meaning; may be synchronous but not synonymous with curing.

Healing Process: a continual journey of changing and evolving of one's self through life; the awareness of patterns that support or are challenges/barriers to health and healing; may be done alone or in a healing community.

Health: the state or process in which the individual (nurse, client, family, group, or community) experiences a sense of well-being, harmony, and unity where subjective experiences about health, health beliefs, and values are honored.

Health Promotion: activities and preventive measures such as immunizations, fitness/exercise programs, breast self exam, appropriate nutrition, relaxation, stress management, social support, prayer, meditation, healing rituals, cultural practices, and promoting environmental health and safety.

Holistic Caring Process: a circular process that involves six steps that may occur simultaneously. These parts are assessment, patterns/problems/needs, outcomes, therapeutic care plan, implementation, and evaluation.

Holistic Communication: a free flow of verbal and nonverbal interchange between and among people and significant beings such as pets, nature, and God/Life Force/Absolute/Transcendent that explores meaning and ideas leading to mutual understanding and growth.

Holistic Nurse: a nurse who recognizes and integrates body-mind-spirit principles and modalities in daily life and clinical practice; one who creates a healing space within herself/himself that allows the nurse to be an instrument of healing for the purpose of helping another feel safe and more in harmony; one who shares authenticity of unconditional presence that helps to remove the barriers to the healing process.

Human Caring Process: the moral state in which the holistic nurse brings her or his whole self into relationship to the whole self of significant beings, which reinforces the meaning and experience of oneness and unity.

Intention: the conscious awareness of being in the present moment to help facilitate the healing process; a volitional act of love.

Intuition: perceived knowing of things and events without the conscious use of rational processes; using all the senses to receive information.

Patterns/Problems/Needs: a person's actual and potential life processes related to health, wellness, disease, or illness that may or may not facilitate well-being.

Person: the concept of person may be defined two ways: (a) a holistic being with interacting subsystems, understanding that the whole is greater than the sum of the parts; (b) an irreducible unitary being.

Person-Centered Care: the condition of trust that is created where holistic care can be given and received; the human caring process in which the holistic nurse gives full attention and intention to the whole self of a person, not merely the current presenting symptoms, illness, crisis, or tasks to be accomplished; reinforcing the person's meaning and experience of communion and unity.

Presence: the essential state or core in healing; approaching an individual in a way that respects and honors her/his essence; relating in a way that reflects a quality of *being with* and *in collaboration with* rather than *doing to*; entering into a shared experience (or field of consciousness) that promotes healing potentials and an experience of well-being.

Spirituality: a unifying force of a person; the essence of being that permeates all of life and is manifested in one's being, knowing, and doing; the interconnectedness with self, others, nature, and God/Life Force/Absolute/Transcendent.

Standards of Practice: a group of statements describing the expected level of care by a holistic nurse.

AHNA HOLISTIC NURSING DESCRIPTION

Holistic nursing embraces all nursing that has enhancement of healing the whole person from birth to death as its goal. Holistic nursing recognizes that there are two views regarding holism: that holism involves identifying the interrelationships of the bio-psycho-social-spiritual dimensions of the person, recognizing that the whole is greater than the sum of its parts; and that holism involves understanding the individual as a unitary whole in mutual process with the environment. Holistic nursing responds to both views, believing that the goals of nursing can be achieved within either framework.

The holistic nurse is an instrument of healing and a facilitator in the healing process. Holistic nurses honor the individual's subjective experience about health, health beliefs, and values. To become therapeutic partners with individuals, families, and communities, holistic nursing practice draws on nursing knowledge, theories, research, expertise, intuition, and creativity. Holistic nursing practice encourages peer review of professional practice in various clinical settings and integrates knowledge of current professional standards, laws, and regulations governing nursing practice.

Practicing holistic nursing requires nurses to integrate self-care, self-responsibility, spirituality, and reflection in their lives. This may lead the nurse to greater awareness of the interconnectedness with self, others, nature, and God/LifeForce/Absolute/Transcendent. This awareness may further enhance the nurses' understanding of all individuals and their relationships to the human and global community, and permits nurses to use this awareness to facilitate the healing process.

INTERVENTIONS MOST FREQUENTLY USED IN HOLISTIC NURSING PRACTICE[1]

Acupressure
Aromatherapy
Art Therapy
Biofeedback
Cognitive Therapy
Counseling[2]
Exercise and Movement
Goal-Setting and Contracts
Guided Imagery
Healing Presence
Healing Touch Modalities
Holistic Self-Assessments
Humor and Laughter
Journaling
Massage
Meditation
Music and Sound Therapy
Nutrition Counseling
Play Therapy
Prayer
Reflexology
Relaxation Modalities
Self-Care Interventions
Self-Reflection
Smoking Cessation
Therapeutic Touch
Weight Management

---

[1]See Dossey, B., Frisch, N., Forker, J., and Lavin, J. Evolving a Blueprint for Certification: Inventory of Professional Activities and Knowledge of a Holistic Nurse, *Journal of Holistic Nursing*, 1998, Vol. 16, No. 1, pp. 33–56.

[2]Used in situations such as addictions, death and grief, unhealthy environments, relationship issues, sexual abuse, spiritual needs, violence, support groups, wellness promotion, and lifestyle issues.

SUMMARY OF AHNA CORE VALUES

Core Value 1. Holistic Philosophy and Education

1.1 Holistic Philosophy: Holistic nurses develop and expand their conceptual framework and overall philosophy in the art and science of holistic nursing to model, practice, teach, and conduct research in the most effective manner possible.

1.2 Holistic Education: Holistic nurses acquire and maintain current knowledge and competency in holistic nursing practice.

Core Value 2. Holistic Ethics, Theories, and Research

2.1 Holistic Ethics: Holistic nurses hold to a professional ethic of caring and healing that seeks to preserve wholeness and dignity of self, students, colleagues, and the person who is receiving care in all practice settings, be it in health promotion, birthing centers, acute or chronic health care facilities, end-of-life care centers, or in homes.

2.2 Holistic Nursing Theories: Holistic nurses recognize that holistic nursing theories provide the framework for all aspects of holistic nursing practice and transformational leadership.

2.3 Holistic Nursing and Related Research: Holistic nurses provide care and guidance to persons through nursing interventions and holistic therapies consistent with research findings and other sound evidence.

Core Value 3. Holistic Nurse Self-Care

3.1 Holistic Nurse Self-Care: Holistic nurses engage in self-care and further develop their own personal awareness of being an instrument of healing to better serve self and others.

Core Value 4. Holistic Communication, Therapeutic Environment, and Cultural Diversity

4.1 Holistic Communication: Holistic nurses engage in holistic communication to ensure that each person experiences the presence of the nurse as authentic and sincere; there is an atmosphere of shared humanness that includes a sense of connectedness and attention reflecting the individual's uniqueness.

4.2 Therapeutic Environment: Holistic nurses recognize that each person's environment includes everything that surrounds the individual, both the external and the internal (physical, mental, emotional, social, and spiritual) as well as patterns not yet understood.

4.3 Cultural Diversity: Holistic nurses recognize each person as a whole body-mind-spirit being and mutually create a plan of care consistent with cultural background, health beliefs, sexual orientation, values, and preferences.

Core Value 5. Holistic Caring Process

5.1 Assessment: Each person is assessed holistically using appropriate traditional and holistic methods while the uniqueness of the person is honored.

5.2 Patterns/Problems/Needs: Actual and potential patterns/ problems/needs and life processes related to health, wellness, disease, or illness which may or may not facilitate well-being are identified and prioritized.

5.3 Outcomes: Each person's actual or potential patterns/problems/ needs have appropriate outcomes specified.

5.4 Therapeutic Care Plan: Each person engages with the holistic nurse to mutually create an appropriate plan of care that focuses on health promotion, recovery or restoration, or peaceful dying so that the person is as independent as possible.

5.5 Implementation: Each person's plan of holistic care is prioritized, and holistic nursing interventions are implemented accordingly.

5.6 Evaluation: Each person's responses to holistic care are regularly and systematically evaluated, and the continuing holistic nature of the healing process is recognized and honored.

AHNA STANDARDS OF HOLISTIC NURSING PRACTICE

CORE VALUE 1. HOLISTIC PHILOSOPHY AND EDUCATION

1.1 Holistic Philosophy: Holistic nurses develop and expand their conceptual framework and overall philosophy in the art and science of holistic nursing to model, practice, teach, and conduct research in the most effective manner possible.

Standards of Practice

Holistic nurses:

1.1.1 recognize the person's capacity for self-healing and the importance of supporting the natural development and unfolding of that capacity.

1.1.2 support, share, and recognize expertise and competency in holistic nursing practice that is used in many diverse clinical and community settings.

1.1.3 participate in person-centered care by being a partner, coach, and mentor who actively listens and supports others in reaching personal goals.

1.1.4 focus on strategies to bring harmony, unity, and healing to the nursing profession.

1.1.5 communicate with traditional health care practitioners about appropriate referrals to other holistic practitioners when needed.

1.1.6 interact with professional organizations in a leadership or membership capacity at local, state, national, and international levels to further expand the knowledge and practice of holistic nursing and awareness of holistic health issues.

1.2 Holistic Education: Holistic nurses acquire and maintain current knowledge and competency in holistic nursing practice.

Standards of Practice

Holistic nurses:

1.2.1 participate in activities of continuing education and related fields that have relevance to holistic nursing practice.

1.2.2 identify areas of knowledge from nursing and various fields such as biomedicine, epidemiology, behavioral medicine, cultural and social theories.

1.2.3 continually develop and standardize holistic nursing guidelines, protocols, and practice to promote competency in holistic nursing practice and assure quality of care to individuals.

1.2.4 use the results of quality care activities to initiate change in holistic nursing practice.

1.2.5 may seek certification in holistic nursing as one means of advancing the philosophy and practice of holistic nursing.

CORE VALUE 2. HOLISTIC ETHICS, THEORIES, AND RESEARCH

2.1 Holistic Ethics: Holistic nurses hold to a professional ethic of caring and healing that seeks to preserve wholeness and dignity of self, students, colleagues, and the person who is receiving care in all practice settings, be it in health promotion, birthing centers, acute or chronic care facilities, end-of-life centers, or homes.

Standards of Practice

Holistic nurses:

2.1.1 identify the ethics of caring and its contribution to unity of self, others, nature, and God/Life Force/Absolute/Transcendent as central to holistic nursing practice.

2.1.2 integrate the standards of holistic nursing practice with applicable state laws and regulations governing nursing practice.

2.1.3 engage in activities that respect, nurture, and enhance the integral relationship with the earth, and advocate for the well-being of the global community's economy, education, and social justice.

2.1.4 advocate for the rights of patients to have educated choices into their plan of care.

2.1.5 participate in peer evaluation to ensure knowledge and competency in holistic nursing practice.

2.1.6 protect the personal privacy and confidentiality of individuals, especially with health care agencies and managed care organizations.

2.2 Holistic Theories: Holistic nurses recognize that holistic nursing theories provide the framework for all aspects of holistic nursing practice and transformational leadership.

Standards of Practice

Holistic nurses:

2.2.1 strive to use nursing theories to develop holistic nursing practice and transformational leadership.

2.2.2 interpret, use, and document information relevant to a person's care according to a theoretical framework.

2.3 Holistic Nursing and Related Research: Holistic nurses provide care and guidance to persons through nursing interventions and holistic therapies consistent with research findings and other sound evidence.

Standards of Practice

Holistic nurses:

2.3.1 use available research and evidence from different explanatory models to mutually create a plan of care with a person.

2.3.2 use expert clinical judgment to select appropriate interventions.

2.3.3 discuss holistic application to clinical situations where rigorous research has not been done.

2.3.4 create an environment conducive to systematic inquiry into healing and health issues by engaging in research or supporting and utilizing the research of others.

2.3.5 disseminate research findings at meetings and through publications to further develop the foundation and practice of holistic nursing.

2.3.6 provide consultation services on holistic nursing interventions to persons and communities based on research.

CORE VALUE 3. HOLISTIC NURSE SELF-CARE

3.1 Holistic Nurse Self-Care: Holistic nurses engage in self-care and further develop their own personal awareness of being an instrument of healing to better serve self and others.

Standards of Practice

Holistic nurses:

3.1.1 recognize that a person's body-mind-spirit has healing capacities that can be enhanced and supported through self-care practices.

3.1.2 identify and integrate self-care strategies to enhance their physical, psychological, sociological, and spiritual well-being.

3.1.3 recognize and address at-risk health patterns and begin the process of change.

3.1.4 consciously cultivate awareness and understanding about the deeper meaning, purpose, inner strengths, and connections with self, others, nature, and God/Life Force/Absolute/Transcendent.

3.1.5 use clear intention to care for self and to seek a sense of balance, harmony, and joy in daily life.

3.1.6 participate in the evolutionary holistic process with the understanding that crisis creates opportunity in any setting.

CORE VALUE 4. HOLISTIC COMMUNICATION, THERAPEUTIC ENVIRONMENT, AND CULTURAL DIVERSITY

4.1 Holistic Communication: Holistic nurses engage in holistic communication to ensure that each person experiences the presence of the nurse as authentic and sincere; there is an atmosphere of shared humanness that includes a sense of connectedness and attention reflecting the individual's uniqueness.

Standards of Practice

Holistic nurses:

4.1.1 develop an awareness of the most frequently encountered challenges to holistic communication.

4.1.2 increase therapeutic and cultural competence skills to enhance their effectiveness through listening to themselves and others.

4.1.3 explore with each person those strategies that can assist her/him, as desired, to understand the deeper meaning, purpose, inner strengths, and connections with self, others, nature, and God/Life Force/ Absolute/Transcendent.

4.1.4 recognize that holistic communication and awareness of individuals is a continuously evolving multi-level exchange that offers itself through dreams, images, symbols, sensations, meditations, and prayers.

4.1.5 respect the person's health trajectory, which may be incongruent with conventional wisdom.

4.2 Therapeutic Environment: Holistic nurses recognize that each person's environment includes everything that surrounds the individual, both the external and internal (physical, mental, emotional, social, and spiritual), as well as patterns not yet understood.

Standards of Practice

Holistic nurses:

4.2.1 promote environments conducive to experiencing healing, wholeness, and harmony, and care for the person in as healthy an environment as possible.

4.2.2 work toward creating organizations that value sacred space and environments that enhance healing.

4.2.3 integrate holistic principles, standards, policies, and procedures in relation to environmental safety and emergency preparedness.

4.2.4 recognize that the well-being of the ecosystem of the planet is a prior determining condition for the well-being of the human.

4.2.5 promote social networks and social environments where healing can take place.

4.3 Cultural Diversity: Holistic nurses recognize each person as a whole being of body-mind-spirit and mutually create a plan of care consistent with cultural backgrounds, health beliefs, sexual orientation, values, and preferences.

Standards of Practice

Holistic nurses:

4.3.1 assess and incorporate the person's cultural practices, values, beliefs, meaning of health, illness, and risk behaviors in care and health education.

4.3.2 use appropriate community resources and experts to extend their understanding of different cultures.

4.3.3 assess for discriminatory practices and change as necessary.

4.3.4 identify discriminatory health care practices as they impact the person and engage in effective nondiscriminatory practices.

CORE VALUE 5. HOLISTIC CARING PROCESS

5.1 Assessment: Each person is assessed holistically using appropriate traditional and holistic methods while the uniqueness of the person is honored.

Standards of Practice

Holistic nurses:

5.1.1 use an assessment process including appropriate traditional and holistic methods to systematically gather information.

5.1.2 value all types of knowing including intuition when gathering data from a person and validate this intuitive knowledge with the person when appropriate.

5.2 Patterns/Problems/Needs: Each person's actual and potential patterns/problems/needs and life processes related to health, wellness, disease, or illness that may or may not facilitate well-being are identified and prioritized.

Standards of Practice

Holistic nurses:

5.2.1 assist the person to access inner wisdom that can provide opportunities to enhance and support growth, development, and movement toward health and well-being.

5.2.2 collect data and collaborate with the person and health care team members as appropriate to identify and record a list of actual and potential patterns/problems/needs.

5.2.3 use collected data to formulate an etiology of the person's identified actual or potential patterns/problems/needs.

5.2.4 make referrals to other holistic practitioners or traditional therapist when appropriate.

5.3 Outcomes: Each person's actual or potential patterns/problems/needs have appropriate outcomes specified.

Standards of Practice

Holistic nurses:

5.3.1 honor the person in all phases of her/his healing process regardless of expectations or outcomes.

5.3.2 identify and partner with the person to specify measurable outcomes and realistic goals.

5.4 Therapeutic Care Plan: Each person engages with the holistic nurse to mutually create an appropriate plan of care that focuses on health promotion, recovery, restoration, or peaceful dying so that the person is as independent as possible.

Standards of Practice

Holistic nurses:

5.4.1 partner with the person in a mutual decision process to create a health care plan for each pattern/problem/need or opportunity to enhance health and well-being.

5.4.2 help a person identify areas for education to make decisions about life choices in a conscious, informed manner that empowers the person to maintain her/his uniqueness and independence.

5.4.3 offer self-assessment tools, word associations, storytelling, dreams, journals as appropriate.

5.4.4 use skills of cultural competence and communicate acceptance of the person's values, beliefs, culture, religion, and socioeconomic background.

5.4.5 assist the person in recognizing at-risk patterns/problems/needs for potential or existing health situations (e.g., personal habits, personal and family health history, age-related risk factors), and also assist in recognizing opportunities to enhance well-being.

5.4.6 engage the person in problem-solving dialogue in relation to living with changes secondary to illness and treatment.

5.5 Implementation: Each person's plan of holistic care is prioritized and holistic nursing interventions are implemented accordingly.

Standards of Practice

Holistic nurses:

5.5.1 implement the mutually created plan of care within the context of assisting the person toward the higher potential of health and well-being.

5.5.2 support and promote the person's capacity for the highest level of participation and problem solving in the plan of care and collaborate with other health team members when appropriate.

5.5.3 use holistic nursing skills in implementing care including cultural competency and all ways of knowing.

5.5.4 advocate that the person's plan, choices, and unique healing journey be honored.

5.5.5 provide care that is clear about and respectful of the economic parameters of practice, balancing justice with compassion.

5.6 Evaluation: Each person's responses to holistic care are regularly and systematically evaluated and the continuing holistic nature of the healing process is recognized and honored.

Standards of Practice

Holistic nurses:

5.6.1 collaborate with the person and with other health care team members when appropriate in evaluating holistic outcomes.

5.6.2 explore with the person her/his understanding of the cause of any significant deviation between the responses and the expected outcomes.

5.6.3 mutually create with the person and other team members a revised plan if needed.

AHNA TASK FORCE

AHNA Task Force Co-Chairpersons

Barbara Montgomery Dossey, MS, RN, HNC, FAAN
Director, Holistic Nursing Consultants
Santa Fe, New Mexico

Noreen Cavan Frisch, PhD, RN, HNC, FAAN
Chair and Professor
Department of Nursing
Cleveland State University
Cleveland, Ohio

AHNA Task Force Committee Members

Cathie E. Guzzetta, PhD, RN, HNC, FAAN
Nursing Research Consultant
Children's Medical Center of Dallas and Parkland Health & Hospital Systems
Director, Holistic Nursing Consultants
Dallas, Texas

Lynn Keegan, PhD, RN, HNC, FAAN
Director, Holistic Nursing Consultants
Port Angeles, Washington

Susan Luck, MA, RN, HNC
Holistic Health Educator
Holistic Nurse Consultant
Director, Nutrition Education
Biodoron Immunology Center
Miami, Florida
Co-Director, Holistic Nursing Associates
New York, New York

Johanne A. Quinn, PhD, RN, HNC
Chair and Professor
Department of Nursing
King College
Bristol, Tennessee

Lynn Rew, EdD, RN, HNC, FAAN
Professor
School of Nursing
The University of Texas at Austin
Austin, Texas

Louise C. Selanders, EdD, RN
Associate Professor
College of Nursing
Michigan State University
East Lansing, Michigan

ADVISORY COMMITTEE MEMBERS

Mary E. Brekke, PhD, RN, HNC, CHTP
Associate Professor
Metropolitan State University
St. Paul, Minnesota
Clinical Specialty: Client Education and Healing Touch

Joanne Evans, MEd, RN, CS, HNC
Psychotherapist, AHNCC Review Board Member
Private Practice
Gaithersburg, Maryland
Clinical Specialty: Psychiatric Clinical Nurse Specialist

Kathleen Fasnacht, MA, MSN, ARNPC, HNC
Geriatric Nurse Practitioner
Bay Pines UAMC
Bay Pines, Florida
Clinical Specialty: Geriatrics

Cheryl Hann, RN, HNC
Private Practice
The Healing Arts Center
Kelowna, BC, Canada
Clinical Specialty: Holistic Nursing

Sharron Harcarik, MS, RN, HNC
Health Education Coordinator
Bristol Park Medical
Irvine, California
Clinical Specialty: Education

Rhonda Kantor, BSN, BS, RN, HNC
President
Global Yoga and Wellness Center
Chicago, Illinois
Clinical Specialty: Home Health Care Specialist

Judy M. Kaplan, BS, RN, CCRC, HNC
Self-employed
Bremerton, Washington
Clinical Specialty: Storytelling and Art Therapy

Kathryn Keegan, RNC, HNC, CHTP
Research Nurse
Veterans Affairs—Connecticut Healthcare System
West Haven, Connecticut
Clinical Specialty: Psychiatry and Substance Abuse

JoAnn Glittenberg Kropp, PhD, RN, HNC, FAAN
Professor of Nursing; Research Professor of Psychiatry and Anthropology
University of Arizona, College of Nursing
Tucson, Arizona
Clinical Specialty: Psychiatric Nursing

Bonnie Mackey, MSN, ARNP, CMT, HNC
Owner and President
Mackey Health Institute, Inc.
Miami, Florida
Clinical Specialty: Adult Holistic Nurse Practitioner, Herbology, Massage & Bodywork

Peggy Moses, MS, RN, MSN
Assistant Professor
Oakton Community College
Des Plaines, Illinois
Clinical Specialty: Education, Administration

Sharon Murnane, BA(c), RN, HNC, CHTP
Holistic Nursing Consultant
Private Practice
San Diego, California
Clinical Specialty: Holistic Nursing

Joyce O. Murphy, BS, RN, HNC
Family Development Coordinator
Western Maine Community Action
Strong, Maine
Clinical Specialty: Community Health Nursing

Laurie Murphy, BSN, RN, HNC
Holistic Nurse
Swedish BodyWorks
Haddam, Connecticut
Clinical Specialty: Healing Energy with Tai Chi and Qi Gong

Bobbie Nisbet, RN, HNC, CHTP
Energy Practitioner
Private Practice
Greensboro, Vermont
Clinical Specialty: Healing Touch, Reiki

Nancy Oliver, PhD, RN, HNC
Associate Professor
California State University
Long Beach, California
Clinical Specialty: Medical/Surgical and Psychosocial Nursing

Clark S. Roberts, RN, HNC, CMT, CHTP
Private Practice
Marquette, Michigan
Clinical Specialty: Wellness Counseling, Massage, Energy Work Practitioner/Instructor

Sonja Simpson, MSN, RN
Executive Director
American Holistic Nurses' Certification Corporation (AHNCC)
Clarkdale, Arizona
Clinical Specialty: Administration/Management

Patricia R. Skidmore, MSN, RN, HNC
Adjunct Faculty
Frederick Community College
Frederick, Maryland
Clinical Specialty: Mental Health

Susanna Smart, BSN, RN, CRT, CMT, CCHT, CRBP, HNC
Biotherapist
Kentfield Rehabilitation Hospital
Private Practice
Kentfield, California
Clinical Specialty: Pain Management/Fibromyalgia

Pina Sperber, BSN, RN
Reiki Practitioner
Chicago, Illinois
Clinical Specialty: Oncology, Reiki

Diane J. Urban, MS, RNC, NP, HNC
Owner/Director
Creative Synergy
Self-employed
Fresno, California
Clinical Specialty: Obstetrics, Women's Health, Home Health, Stress Management

Christine B. Ussard, BSN, RN, HNC
Clinical Coordinator
Orleans Anesthesia Group
New Orleans, Louisiana
Clinical Specialty: Pain Management

Gretchen Wiederrecht, MS, RN, HNC
Nurse Therapist
Senior Outreach Team Montgomery County
Silver Spring, Maryland
Clinical Specialty: Psychiatry

REVIEW COMMITTEE

Jeanne Anselmo, BSN, RN, HNC
Holistic Nurse Consultant
Private Practice
New York, New York
Clinical Specialty: Holistic Nursing, Wellness Healthcare Consulting

Elizabeth Ann Manhart Barrett, PhD, RN, FAAN
Professor and Coordinator
Center for Nursing Research
Hunter College, City University of New York
New York, New York
Clinical Specialty: Mental Health

Genevieve M. Bartol, EdD, RN, HNC
Professor Emeritus
University of North Carolina at Greensboro
Greensboro, North Carolina
Clinical Specialty: Psychiatric/Mental Health Nursing

Margaret A. Burkhardt, PhD, RN, CS, HNC
Associate Professor & Family Nurse Practitioner
West Virginia University School of Nursing
Charleston, West Virginia
Clinical Specialty: Holistic Nursing, Family Nurse Practitioner

Nancy Fleming Courts, PhD, RN, NCC
Associate Professor and Chair
University of North Carolina at Greensboro
Greensboro, North Carolina
Clinical Specialty: Adult Health

Joan Engebretson, DrPH, RN, HNC
Associate Professor
University of Texas Health Science Center at Houston School of Nursing
Houston, Texas
Clinical Specialty: Maternal-Child Health and Women's Health Care

Kimetha S. Falkenburg, BSN, RN
Staff Nurse
Central Baptist Hospital
Lexington, Kentucky
Clinical Specialty: Critical Care

Lea Barbato Gaydos, PhD, MSN, RN, CS, HNC
Director
Beth-El College of Nursing
Holistic Nursing Studies
University of Colorado at Colorado Springs
Colorado Springs, Colorado
Clinical Specialty: Holistic Nursing and Community Psychiatric Mental Health Nursing

Dorothea Hover-Kramer, EdD, RN
Director
Behavior Health Consultants
Private Practice
Poway, California
Clinical Specialty: Bereavement Counseling, Energy Healing with Healing Touch, Pandimensional Balancing

Pamela J. Potter Hughes, MSN, RNCS, CHTP/I
Doctoral Student
Yale University
New Haven, Connecticut
Director and Practitioner
New Haven Center for Nursing Therapeutics
New Haven, Connecticut
Clinical Specialty: Adult Mental Health/Psychiatric Nursing and Psychoenergetic Therapy

Mary Gail Nagai Jacobson, MSN, RN
Community Health Consultant
San Marcos, Texas
Clinical Specialty: Psychiatric Mental Health Nursing and Hospice

Karen Kauffeld, RN
Clinical Coordinator
Mind-Body Wellness Center
Meadville, Pennsylvania
Clinical Specialty: Holistic Nursing, and Complementary and Alternative Therapies

Cheryl Demerath Learn, PhD, RN
Associate Professor
College of Nursing
Health Sciences Center
University of New Mexico
Albuquerque, New Mexico
Clinical Specialty: Women, Aging and Health

Maggie McKivergin, MS, RN, CNS, HNC
Holistic Nurse Consultant
Nurse Coordinator
Center for Alternative Health Care Practitioners, Inc.
Charleston, West Virginia
Clinical Specialty: Holistic Nursing

Melodie Olson, PhD, RN
Associate Professor
College of Nursing, Medical University of South Carolina
Charleston, South Carolina
Clinical Specialty: Adult Health

B.H. Rose, MEd, MSN, RN
City of Austin Health and Human Services
Austin, Texas
Clinical Specialty: Public Health

Bonney Gulino Schaub, MS, RN, CS
Director of Clinical Imagery and Meditation
New York Psychosynthesis Institute
New York, New York
Clinical Specialty: Adult Psychiatric Mental Health Nursing, Psychotherapy Practice, Education and Consultation in Holistic Practice

Eleanor A. Schuster, DNSc, RN, HNC
Professor
College of Nursing, Florida Atlantic University
Boca Raton, Florida
Clinical Specialty: Family-Based Holistic Nursing

Eileen M. Stuart, RN, MS
Cardiovascular Nurse Practitioner
WellCare Associates
Boston, Massachusetts
Clinical Specialty: Cardiovascular and Wellness Counseling

Leona Weiner, EdD, RN, HNC
Professor Emeritus
Long Island University, Division of Nursing
New York, New York
Clinical Specialty: Pediatrics, Community Health Education, Mental Health Consultation

Carol L. Wells-Federman, MS, MEd, RN, CS
Co-Director Chronic Pain Management Program
Beth Israel Deaconess Hospital
Boston, Massachusetts
Clinical Specialty: Chronic Pain Management

Wendy Wetzel, MSN, RN, FNP, HNC
Nurse Practitioner
Private Practice
Flagstaff, Arizona
Clinical Specialty: Women's Health

Patty Wooten, BSN, RN
Nurse-Humorist
Jest for the Health of It
Santa Cruz, California
Clinical Specialty: Humor and Laughter Therapy

Christine A. Wynd, PhD, RN
Professor of Nursing
University of Akron
Akron, Ohio
Clinical Specialty: Health Promotion

LEADERSHIP COMMITTEE*

Linda Chiofar, MA, RN, HNC
Holistic Health Nurse
Center for Well Being
San Leandro, California
Clinical Specialty: Wellness Practice/Educator

Jeanne Colbath, RN, MSN, ANP, HNC
AHNA Northeast Regional Director
St. Elizabeth's Medical Center
Boston, Massachusetts
Clinical Specialty: Cardiovascular Rehabilitation

Sue Collins, MEd, MSN, RN, CFNP, HNC
Clinical Director
North Community Health Center
Flagstaff, Arizona
Clinical Specialty: Family Nurse Practitioner

Charlotte Eliopoulos, PhD, RNC
Specialist in Holistic Geriatric and Chronic Care Nursing
Health Education Network
Glen Arm, Maryland
Clinical Specialty: Gerontological Nursing, Long-Term Care Nursing

*The Leadership Committee was composed of AHNA Leadership Council Members that responded to the AHNA Standards Task Force Committee.

Linda C. Gallagher, MPH, BSN, RN
Certified Diabetes Educator—CDC HT Practitioner-CHTP
Health Promotion Consultant, Healing Touch
Practitioner, Self-employed
Media, Pennsylvania
Clinical Specialty: Holistic Health Program Planning and Development, Healing Touch Practitioner

Eve Karpinski, BSN, BA, RNC, HNC
Program Director
Shore Line Behavioral Health
Toms River, New Jersey
Clinical Specialty: Psychiatric and Mental Health

Judy A. Koenig, BSN, RN
AHNA North Central Regional Director
Staff Nurse
Veterans Affairs Medical Center
Omaha, Nebraska
Clinical Specialty: Surgical Intensive Care

Diane Pisanos, MS, RNC, NNP, HNC
Neonatal Nurse Practitioner and Private Consultant
Presbyterian St. Luke's Medical Center
Denver, Colorado
Clinical Specialty: Neonatal Nurse Practitioner

Karilee Halo Shames, PhD, RN, HNC
Director, Nurse Empowerment Workshops & Services
Assistant Professor
College of Nursing
Florida Atlantic University
Boca Raton, Florida
Clinical Specialty: Psychiatric Nursing and Holistic Practice

Lori Wyzykowski, RN, CHTP/I, HNC
Private Practice
West Palm Beach, Florida
Clinical Specialty: Healing Touch/Holistic Nursing Educator

CORE VALUE 1

HOLISTIC PHILOSOPHY AND EDUCATION

Noreen Cavan Frisch

1.1 Holistic Philosophy

■■ Holistic nurses develop and expand their conceptual framework and overall philosophy in the art and science of holistic nursing to model, practice, teach, and conduct research in the most effective manner possible. ■■

Holistic philosophy, as the first Core Value, provides the foundation for a nurse's practice. A philosophy is defined as "the system which a person forms for the conduct of life; the mental attitude or habit of the person."[1] For many, philosophy represents a search for meaning. In the discipline of nursing, a philosophy of nursing represents one's beliefs about the profession that provide a perspective for practice, scholarship, and research.[2] Holistic nurses share a philosophy based on a perspective that acknowledges and values the connectedness of the body-mind-spirit, the inherent goodness of human beings, the ability of each person to find meaning and purpose in his or her own life, and the nurse's role of support to each client so that the client may find comfort, peace, and harmony. Holistic nurses practice from a perspective that comprehends both the art and science of the profession: thus, nursing practice is simultaneously "right- and left-brained." Holistic nurses live professional and personal lives that expand their knowledge and understanding of human beings, of nursing, and of themselves. The original use of the term philosophy in the English language is the widest sense of the word—"the love, study, or pursuit of wisdom, or of knowledge of things and their causes."[1] Applied to the philosophy of nursing, this definition connotes the joy of learning, understanding, and living that is an essential core of holistic practice. There are six Standards of Practice that demonstrate the Core Value of philosophy; each is described and illustrated in the pages that follow.

Standard of Practice 1.1.1

Holistic nurses recognize the person's capacity for self-healing and the importance of supporting the natural development and unfolding of that capacity.

This Standard underscores the value holistic nurses place on self-healing and self-determination of the client. Further, the nursing role in supporting a natural developmental process of growth is emphasized. Use of the term "unfolding" represents the unfolding or mystery of the human spirit. The Standard dictates that the nurse comprehend the basic capacity or power of each individual receiving nursing care and act to support the natural progression, movement, or evolution inherent within each individual. Table 1–1 illustrates the nursing knowledge and skill required for a nurse to meet this Standard.

Table 1–1 Self-Healing

Standard of Practice 1.1.1	*Key Concepts*	*Requisite Knowledge*	*Requisite Skills*
Holistic nurses recognize the person's capacity for self-healing and the importance of supporting the natural development and unfolding of that capacity.	Capacity for self-healing. Natural development. Unfolding of human capacity.	Scientific knowledge of healing, recovery. Developmental theories that explain phenomena of growth, change, and maturation. Knowledge of the inherent movement or evolution of the human spirit; comprehension of the mystery of human life.	Ability to study, reflect, and gain knowledge. Interpersonal communication skills through which the nurse can demonstrate support to another. Healing presence, empathy, installation of hope. Ability to reflect a positive orientation to others and to self.

Nursing Activities

Nursing actions that demonstrate this Standard include: healing presence, caring/nurturance, promotion of positive regard, empathy, and installation of hope.

Healing presence is the ability of the nurse to provide each client with an interpersonal encounter that is experienced as the presence of one who is giving undivided attention to the needs and concerns of the client in a manner that is positive, supportive, and loving.[3] Caring/nurturance is the expression of true regard for the client, coupled with the performance of nursing activities required for care.[4] Promotion of positive regard is a reflection of the basic belief in the goodness of people and the ability to convey to the client the belief in *his or her* worth and value as a human being.[4] Empathy is the ability to understand the world from the client's perspective and feel the subjective experience of another.[4] Installation of hope is the ability to support each person in developing a positive outlook and searching for a meaning and purpose in life.[5]

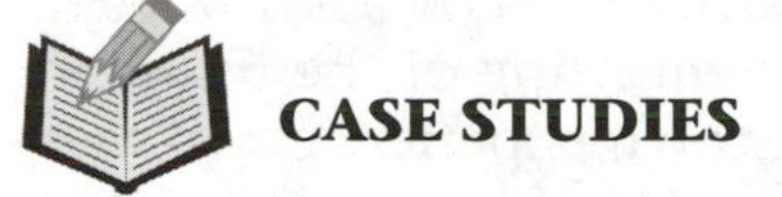

CASE STUDIES

1 Nurse MaryAnne was working in a trauma center as Joe was brought in after a car accident. Joe had multiple injuries—probable fracture of the ribs and wrist, lacerations to the face, and a broken tooth. Joe expressed pain, difficulty in breathing, and fear residual to the experience of having his car hit by another vehicle. He was alert and oriented. MaryAnne needed to obtain a brief history of the accident, take vital signs, and perform a nursing assessment of his condition. In so doing, MaryAnne expressed an awareness of Joe as an individual, expressed her concern that she wished to meet his needs, and provided support and reassurance to Joe that the hospital staff were there to help. She gently touched his shoulder and said "Car accidents are usually frightening experiences. We are here to assess whatever injuries you have and to give you care. I will be with you during your treatment here. Tell me anything that you think we should know about you." Her manner was sincere, her movements were unhurried, and her being was fully present.

In this example, MaryAnne is practicing the Standard of support to the individual with belief in his ability and capacity for self-healing. While the hospital staff know how to care for fractures and lacerations, she acknowledges that they don't know how to care for *Joe.* He needs to tell her that.

Nursing Tip:

How can a busy nurse be fully present?

How can a nurse in a trauma center demonstrate movements that are perceived as unhurried?

Every nurse must wash his or her hands before giving care to clients. As part of this routine handwashing, think of the washing of your hands as a cleansing of your mind. As you wash your hands, take a deep breath and clear your mind and being so that you can be ready to accept a new human being into your care.

2 Nurse Beverly was working in an oncology unit. Her client, Mrs. Anderson, had breast cancer and was hospitalized following a lumpectomy. Mrs. Anderson was scheduled to have chemotherapy over the next few weeks. Mrs. Anderson had read much information about her condition and had discussed various options for treatment with her family physician, her oncologist, and her nurse. She had given fully informed consent for her treatments. She was also following a diet prescribed in a popular best-selling book. When Beverly approached her client, Mrs. Anderson appeared distracted. Even though Beverly only had five minutes at this time, Beverly sat down and questioned Mrs. Anderson about her needs and concerns. Beverly said, "What are your worries and wants?" Mrs. Anderson only replied that she wasn't sure of her future. Beverly listened and rephrased the statement, "You're not sure of your future?"

In using the communication technique of rephrasing, Beverly acknowledges she heard, does not jump to conclusions about the meaning of the future for her client, and invites Mrs. Anderson to explore her own experience and share it with her nurse. By sitting down, she brings a presence of true concern. Beverly's actions are consistent with Standard 1.1.1 because she provides individual care, based on concern about the client's subjective feelings and sense of what will or what can happen. In the conversation that followed, Beverly formed the basis for a nurse-client interaction that could explore and support Mrs. Anderson's sense of meaning and purpose.

3 Nurse Nancy was providing care in a university student health center. She was taking a history from a young woman, Marie, who came to the health center with concerns over flu-like symptoms. Nancy took the immediate history and proceeded to provide appropriate treatment recommendations. She gave her client a handout on self-care for her symptoms, and assessed that Marie understood the recommendations.

While Nancy's care is appropriate and professional, in this situation Nancy does not demonstrate compliance with Standard 1.1.1. There is nothing in Nancy's care that acknowledged Marie as an individual, nor did she assess the meaning of the illness to Marie at this particular time.

Standard of Practice 1.1.2

Holistic nurses support, share, and recognize expertise and competency in holistic nursing practice that is used in many diverse clinical and community settings.

This Standard refers to practice on several levels. First, the nurse must understand that there is a continuum of care environments wherein nursing is practiced. Nursing care settings are not restricted to hospitals or clinics, or even to clients' homes. Care environments extend to private offices, nursing homes and skilled nursing facilities, clinics, community centers, churches and places of worship, schools, and locations of a myriad of support groups. Further, a care environment can be made through telephone or even Internet contact with another. The telephone provides a quick access for communication between nurse and client. As part of setting up an environment of caring and response, nurses can ensure that clients have a phone number where the nurse can be reached.With more and more people communicating on the Internet, there is an increasing number of discussion groups related to specific illnesses. Some nurses have set up closed discussion groups for certain clients, and many nurses accept e-mail communications. Holistic nurses recognize competency in holistic nursing practice wherever and however it takes place, and take steps to support that practice. Further, holistic nurses share their experiences with other nurses so as to assist others in being successful. Lastly, holistic nurses, in sharing competency in holistic nursing, will take steps to publicize nursing success in practice, where appropriate. Table 1–2 illustrates the nursing knowledge and skill needed to meet Standard 1.1.2.

Table 1–2 Expertise and Competency in Holistic Nursing

Standard of Practice 1.1.2	*Key Concepts*	*Requisite Knowledge*	*Requisite Skills*
Holistic nurses support, share, and recognize expertise and competency in holistic nursing practice that is used in many diverse clinical and community settings.	Support, share, and recognize expertise and competence in holistic nursing. Diverse clinical and community settings.	Understanding of and experience with a variety of nursing care environments. Knowledge of data analysis that supports competency in practice.	Ability to provide professional support and/or mentoring to other nurses. Communication skills—both oral and written—to share with other nurses, and the community at large, the accomplishments of holistic nursing.

Nursing Activities

Nursing activities that demonstrate this Standard include: actions that nurses take to support and nurture other nurses; the critical thinking required to recognize competency in nursing practice; and communication techniques that allow nurses to share, both orally and in writing, the accomplishments of holistic nursing. Nurses often have the choice of supporting other nurses, or not. And, as a profession, nurses are not known for their ability to accept new nurses or new ideas into practice settings. Support and nurturance of others' attempts to provide holistic care require a willingness to praise others for their accomplishments, efforts, and any actions taken in the work setting to give nurses the chance to incorporate alternative models into their care. Ability to distinguish competent holistic practice from practice that is not requires nurses to study the Standards of Holistic Nursing Practice to know when practice is in compliance with these Standards. Sharing the results of holistic nursing care demands that the nurse speak in a manner such that communication can be heard and understood. For example, the holistic nurse must be able to speak to a room full of physicians at a case conference, a family group asking questions about care, a newspaper reporter doing a story on a new community clinic, and representatives of a State Board of Nursing. The language used will be quite different for each group—in order to fully support and share expertise and competency in holistic practice, the nurse must be able to change his or her manner of communication so that diverse groups understand the communication.

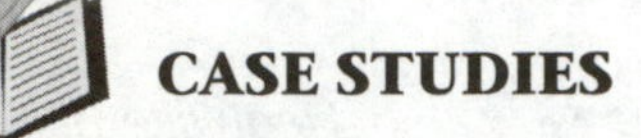

CASE STUDIES

1 Nurse Ralph was in charge of school nursing for a major metropolitan school district. One of the nurses he supervises, Grace, came to him with a proposal to open a community clinic at a high school that would be open to the high school students and their families. There was a possibility of grant funding for the project. As Ralph talked with Grace about her plan, she explained that the nurse-run clinic could offer alternative and complementary modalities along with health education efforts aimed at the priority needs of the client population. These priority needs included care of upper respiratory illnesses, reducing the number of accidental injuries such as injuries at school, attention to the issue of depression in the teenage population, and information related to reproductive health and sexuality. Grace provided data on the use of folk treatments for respiratory illnesses common among persons in the school community. She also provided information on the appropriateness of diet and nutritional supplements that were consistent with the practices of her clients. Ralph saw that the data were anecdotal; however, he knew that there was reason to believe Grace wasn't wrong in her conclusions. To support the idea of a nurse-run clinic and the possibility of providing care that is sensitive to the practices of the school community, he worked with Grace to conduct a needs assessment. Further, he helped Grace obtain research data published in the nursing and health literature about the nutritional interventions she was proposing.

In this example, Ralph recognizes a sincere attempt to meet clients' needs, values Grace's innovation and plans, and uses his abilities to assist her to bring her proposal to the point where it meets the Standards of Holistic Nursing Practice, and also where grant funding is more probable. He worked with Grace, giving her credit for the idea while he supported her to meet standards of competency. Ralph's behaviors are in compliance with Standard 1.1.2.

2 Mary is a nurse in a same-day surgi-center. One of her colleagues, Tim, brought forth a proposal to incorporate the use of guided imagery into the policy and procedure manual of the center. Tim provided data on the use of guided imagery in surgical clients and discussed research indicating that at least some clients are comforted through the use of this technique. As Tim described his plan to her, Mary expressed her belief that the plan was competent. When Tim took his proposal to upper administration, Mary remained silent and decided to wait until someone contacted her for her opinion. While she recognized the value and competency of the proposal, she did not show support nor did she share in the opportunity to publicly articulate the reason for or value of a holistic nursing approach. There is nothing wrong with Mary's actions as a professional nurse, but she did not demonstrate actions in keeping with Standard 1.1.2.

Standard of Practice 1.1.3

Holistic nurses participate in person-centered care by being a partner, coach, and mentor who actively listens and supports others in reaching personal goals.

This Standard emphasizes the nurse's role as a facilitator and support person, and as one who is engaged in an interpersonal relationship with the client of nursing. Holistic nursing philosophy suggests that the nurse must never objectify the client (i.e., treat the client as an object). The nurse is required to come to the client encounter ready to meet and assist a unique human being. To truly help another person (or a group of persons), the nurse must learn of the client's perspectives and personal goals. The nurse, as one who has health-related knowledge and skills, must use these skills to assist the client to make personal choices that are health directed. The relationship between the client and nurse is one of a partner or trusted coach/mentor. The nurse never takes on an authoritarian role; rather, the nurse maintains the client's dignity at all times by ensuring that the nurse-client relationship is one of person-to-person interaction and support.

Table 1–3 summarizes this Standard.

Table 1–3 Person-Centered Care

Standard of Practice 1.1.3	*Key Concepts*	*Requisite Knowledge*	*Requisite Skills*
Holistic nurses participate in person-centered care by being a partner, coach, and mentor who actively listens and supports others in reaching personal goals.	Person-centered care. Partner, coach, mentor. Active listening. Support for others.	Knowledge of how persons are alike and how persons are different. Knowledge of nursing roles of facilitator and support-person. Nursing knowledge of health, illness, and wellness to assist others to achieve personal health-related goals.	Ability to empathize and to see and understand the world from another's perspective. Interpersonal skills of communication and offering support. Ability to engage in a significant human relationship.

Nursing Activities

Nursing activities consistent with this Standard include empathic communication and establishing a presence that facilitates trust. A nurse must have the client's trust for the nurse and client to be able to engage in a significant therapeutic relationship. The client must be willing to disclose his or her health and life goals and be willing to examine various methods of achieving those goals with the nurse. Trust in the nurse can also assist the client to trust *his or her* own plans to achieve goals.

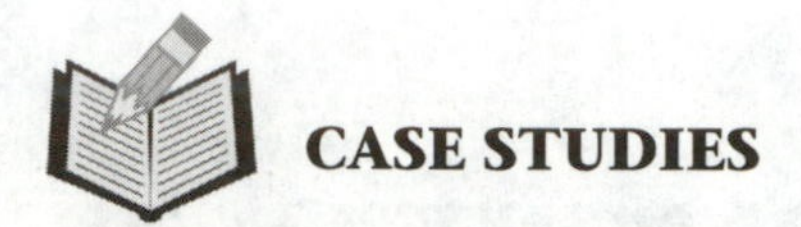

CASE STUDIES

1 Nurse Emily was caring for an elderly woman, Mrs. McCann, in an Adult Day Health Center. The woman came for rehabilitation after a mild stroke. Mrs. McCann had been referred to the Center by hospital staff and her private physician. The Center's activity director scheduled Mrs. McCann for several activities during the day including a chair-based exercise group, time in physical therapy, a socialization group, and time in the Center's library/computer room. Emily greeted Mrs. McCann and her daughter on their arrival the first day and asked them both to meet with her to discuss the Center's offerings and Mrs. McCann's needs and wants. Upon discussion, Emily learned that Mrs. McCann is a quiet person and had never engaged in group activities in her life. Mrs. McCann stated that she sees physical therapy exercise as the most important reason for her participation at the Center. Mrs. McCann further stated that her goal was to regain her sense of balance and return her confidence in her own physical abilities. Emily then worked with Mrs. McCann to identify how she could spend her day to work toward accomplishing her own goals, making herself comfortable at the Center. Her daily schedule was changed to include more time in the library/computer room, time twice a week in the Center's swimming pool, and less time in group activities.

2 Nurse Molly worked in the same Adult Day Health Center. Mr. Kirk came to the Center the same day as Mrs. McCann. Molly checked the referral papers from Mr. Kirk's physician. He had been referred after a mild stroke as well. His physician and physical therapist recommended a series of exercises. Molly brought Mr. Kirk into the daily activities (physical therapy, chair exercise, socialization group, and library). Molly provided an excellent orientation to the Center and to its activities.

In the case examples described above, Emily is providing care consistent with the Standard 1.1.3, and Molly is not. Emily is approaching her client as a unique human being and takes the time to learn of Mrs. McCann's individual needs and wants. Molly is providing care expected by the Center, but she is failing to recognize Mr. Kirk as an individual and is not making accommodation to any individual needs he may have.

Standard of Practice 1.1.4

Holistic nurses focus on strategies to bring harmony, unity, and healing to the nursing profession.

There are many reasons why holistic nurses must take steps to heal their profession. Nursing is at a crossroads, being pulled in many directions by persons and stakeholders who have the ability to make demands on nurses and dictate conditions of nursing's work. Nurses, under stress from factors external to themselves (for example, managed care), have not responded as a united group of professionals seeking the best for their clients and their profession. On an individual basis, many nurses are not supportive of the new nurses coming into the profession or supportive of others' career paths. On a state and national level, leadership positions within nursing are open for nurses who can help to move the profession forward while at the same time providing collaboration (rather than competition) and support for others.

Holistic nurses have a responsibility to take a leadership role in any activity that promotes health and healing of nursing. The AHNA Code of Ethics for Holistic Nursing Practice specifically states that "nurses have a responsibility to nurture each other."[6] Holistic nurses celebrate the accomplishments of every nurse. Table 1–4 illustrates the concepts, knowledge, and skills required by Standard 1.1.4.

Table 1–4 Harmony, Unity, and Healing to the Nursing Profession

Standard of Practice 1.1.4	*Key Concepts*	*Requisite Knowledge*	*Requisite Skills*
Holistic nurses focus on strategies to bring harmony, unity, and healing to the nursing profession.	Healing to the nursing profession.	Knowledge of various career paths for nurses. Knowledge of the effectiveness of collective action.	Nurturance and caring for other nurses. Political action and advocacy.

Nursing Activities

The nursing activities that are consistent with this Standard include activities in two areas: those that support other nurses and those that support the nursing profession.

To support other nurses, every nurse must be as kind and compassionate toward coworkers as one is toward clients. Holistic nurses recognize that new nurses need mentors, grow from encouragement, and require a supportive working environment. Measures that assist other nurses include using self as mentor to others, being a "team player" in any workgroup, and taking time to notice and comment upon other nurses' accomplishments and good work.

To support the nursing profession, the holistic nurse joins nursing organizations, either specialty associations or national organizations such as the American Nurses Association, for the purpose of supporting nursing as a whole. Further, the nurse stands ready to speak out about nursing on a local, regional, or national level to portray a positive nursing point of view to the public. Lastly, holistic nurses identify their work as *Nursing* and embrace the professional practice of nursing.

CASE STUDIES

1 Cathy, an experienced nurse with over 10 years of practice in medical-surgical nursing and critical care, was working in a suburban hospital. She was comfortable in her ability to practice on any of the floors at the facility giving care to adult patients. Charlotte, a new nurse who recently passed NCLEX, was hired to work on the medical-surgical unit of the floors. Charlotte was eager to put into practice all of the skills she had learned; she was motivated to work hard and be a good nurse. When Cathy came to work one day, she was assigned to work on the same unit as Charlotte. After report, Cathy said to Charlotte: "Welcome to our hospital. I know you are new here, so don't hesitate to ask me if you can't find something or don't know our routines—I've been here a while so I probably can help." Cathy's remark was done with the recognition that she had a duty to help new nurses. Further, Cathy knew that once she offered help, she would have to spend some of her time with Charlotte, answering questions, and organizing her own time to "take care of" another new nurse.

Cathy is able to accept her role in bringing another person successfully into nursing. Cathy's actions are in keeping with Standard 1.1.4 because she is reaching out to a new nurse. She is supporting the newcomer and approaches Charlotte in a manner of acceptance. Cathy is aware of the fact that Charlotte is a novice nurse, and that she, as an experienced and competent nurse, has an obligation to support others. Cathy's actions help to bring unity to the nursing profession.

2 Laverne is a holistic nurse working in oncology. She joined the AHNA because she wants to learn about new developments in holistic nursing and in complementary care. She also joined the Oncology Nursing Society so she can keep abreast of developments in cancer care and treatments. When she attended a meeting of regional oncology nurses, she found that many of the oncology nurses were unaware of the specialty of holistic nursing. Then, when her local oncology nurses' group decided to form a committee to evaluate the control of pain in terminal cancer patients, she volunteered to serve. Laverne believed that through work on this committee, she could open up some new ideas for others and introduce them to some modalities and concepts used by holistic nurses.

Laverne serves as a "bridge" between two specialties. She is meeting Standard 1.1.4 because she is bringing knowledge and skills from one nursing specialty to another. Laverne is helping to bring unity to two groups of nurses, assisting them to see their similarities and common interests.

Standard of Practice 1.1.5

Holistic nurses communicate with traditional health care practitioners about appropriate referrals to other holistic practitioners when needed.

Holistic nurses provide information about the practice of other holistic nurses and holistic practitioners to traditional care providers in the interest of advancing knowledge about holistic care and advocating for the best and most comprehensive client care possible. The knowledge possessed by holistic nurses can and should be shared so that those providers who have limited information on services available, or on services that their clients use, can be informed. The holistic nurse serves as a professional contact for others. Table 1–5 summarizes the concepts, knowledge, and skills required by Standard 1.1.5.

Table 1–5 Communication with Health Care Practitioners

Standard of Practice 1.1.5	*Key Concepts*	*Requisite Knowledge*	*Requisite Skills*
Holistic nurses communicate with traditional health care practitioners about appropriate referrals to other holistic practitioners when needed.	Professional communication. Client referrals.	Referral networks in one's community.	Professional credibility. Interdisciplinary communication.

Nursing Activities

Nursing activities that demonstrate this Standard include: compiling a network in one's own community of holistic nurses and other holistic health care providers; observing client behaviors and actions to assess when referrals are appropriate; and maintaining credibility with traditional health care providers so that professional communication regarding referrals can occur.

CASE STUDY

1 Nurse May worked in a public health department. One of her new assignments was to assist a community social worker in his running of a support group for members of the urban community who are individuals living with HIV or AIDS. May attended the support group and observed several persons telling their stories of living in fear, some of whom were also living in physical pain. Many other members of the group reported having lost weight and energy. One person in the group expressed feelings of social isolation and being cut off and removed from others. Jose, the social worker, provided an atmosphere in the group of support, acceptance, and problem solving.

After the group meeting, May approached Jose and provided him with information about many of the holistic health providers she knew in the community. These included holistic nurses who practice therapeutic touch, healing touch, and guided imagery; nurses who were certified in massage therapy; a music therapist; and volunteers who ran a program in pet-assisted therapy. May asked Jose if he thought the group attendees would benefit from these modalities. Jose was interested in the idea but questioned the credibility of the practitioners. May was able to describe the level of expertise among the practitioners she had suggested, knowing that each carried certification from a national organization. May also described the research behind the modalities and suggested that the support group of clients may have interest in knowing about these practitioners. Jose agreed, and for the next group session, May described the holistic practitioners in the community, and the clients began to think about whether or not they wished to be referred.

May's behaviors are in keeping with Standard 1.1.5. Not only did May have the information about the holistic providers, but she also knew how to approach Jose, her colleague, and provide him with information and evidence of credible practice. May then provided the information and the option for referral to the clients. Not only did May make sure that the clients knew about the services, but she educated a colleague about the services as well.

Standard of Practice 1.1.6

Holistic nurses interact with professional organizations in a leadership or membership capacity at local, state, national, and international levels to further expand the knowledge and practice of holistic nursing and awareness of holistic health issues.

This Standard underscores that holistic nurses stand ready to assume leadership roles in the profession of nursing for the purpose of advancing holism. Holistic nurses are encouraged to join organizations in their nursing specialty, as well as joining AHNA. Further, the AHNA and any group of holistic nurses are encouraged to support members in developing leadership skills.

Nursing Activities

Activities that demonstrate compliance with this Standard include joining organizations, determining the degree to which one can be active in each, prioritizing time to make organizational participation meaningful, and serving each group in a capacity that is supportive and advances holistic ideals. Meaningful participation in any organization includes following through on all commitments, working for the benefit of the collective, and being equally comfortable leading or following as the situation demands.

Table 1–6 summarizes Standard 1.1.6.

Table 1–6 Professional Organizations

Standard of Practice 1.1.6	*Key Concepts*	*Requisite Knowledge*	*Requisite Skills*
Holistic nurses interact with professional organizations in a leadership or membership capacity at local, state, national, and international levels to further expand the knowledge and practice of holistic nursing and awareness of holistic health issues.	Interact with professional organizations. Expand knowledge and awareness of holism.	Knowledge of nursing and specialty organizations.	Skills of organizational membership, including skills of leadership and followership.

CASE STUDIES

1 Linda is a nurse who was a member of the Pediatric Nursing Association, the Society of Rogerian Scholars, Sigma Theta Tau, and the AHNA. She was interested in all of these groups but found she was unable to attend regular meetings of each. She worked as a pediatric nurse and believed that the materials she received from the Pediatric group were most helpful in keeping up to date in her immediate work. She decided that she must participate at a regional and national level in pediatric care. However, she discovered through reading a newsletter that there were several nurses in the Rogerian Society that were interested in applications of this holistic theory to children and their families. Linda volunteered to work with these nurses in a study group and ultimately decided to use her practice in a pilot project related to the theory. While Linda kept her membership in the other groups, she decided to focus on two organizations and participate actively.

Linda's actions are in keeping with Standard 1.1.6. She manages her time well to prioritize how she can best make a contribution and develop her own work. She is interacting with her professional organizations in a contributory and responsible way.

2 Wendy is a member of AHNA and active in her local network. She learned that her State Nurses Association (SNA), affiliated with ANA, was having a meeting in her home town. She called her AHNA networker and asked if she could help to bring a presence of holistic nursing to the SNA meeting. She and the networker talked about how to set up a booth to display AHNA philosophy and resources. Wendy then approached the SNA meeting planners and made arrangements to represent AHNA at the meeting.

Wendy attended the SNA meeting as the official representative of AHNA. Wendy discovered that many nurses were interested in holism and, after a day of working at the booth, she became a designated liaison between the two groups. Wendy was asked to attend the next meeting of SNA as a speaker on holistic resources in her state.

Wendy's actions are in keeping with Standard 1.1.6. She takes initiative, represents AHNA with the help and support of her networker, and develops herself as the liaison between two groups.

1.2 Holistic Education

■■ Holistic nurses acquire and maintain current knowledge and competency in holistic nursing practice. ■■

A Core Value emphasizing *education* draws attention to the need for lifelong learning and professional growth and development over the time of one's career. Like many revisions that will undoubtedly transform the 21st century, the changes impacting health care will be profound. Research data on the use and effects of various treatments are published almost daily, and such information is immediately available to practitioners through computerized databases. All nurses must keep up with current knowledge to maintain safe and legally defensible practice. In order to take on leadership roles in the profession, holistic nurses must ensure that they are current in the specialty of holistic care, and must maintain currency with developments in nursing, nursing theory, and organization of nursing services. Continuing education, whether in the form of continuing education classes, academic courses, or self-study, helps the nurse to understand the changing context in which care is delivered, as well as helping the nurse to consider new knowledge and understandings of nursing interventions. There are five Standards of Practice that demonstrate the Core Value of education; each is described and illustrated in the section that follows.

Standard of Practice 1.2.1

Holistic nurses participate in activities of continuing education and related fields that have relevance to holistic nursing practice.

This Standard presents an expectation that holistic nurses seek out educational offerings, both in nursing (those activities for which continuing education credit is offered) and in related fields that may have direct impact on the nurses' practice. The Standard does not specify the content of such continuing education, for there is an expectation that the nurse can identify which activities best support his or her practice. The Standard is that continuing education be an ongoing activity, one that the nurse recognizes is a requirement to keep one's practice and care at the professional level. Table 1–7 summarizes Standard 1.2.1.

Table 1–7 Continuing Education

Standard of Practice 1.2.1	*Key Concepts*	*Requisite Knowledge*	*Requisite Skills*
Holistic nurses participate in activities of continuing education and related fields that have relevance to holistic nursing practice.	Participation in continuing education. Nursing and related fields.	Knowledge of trends in the discipline and area of practice. Knowledge of continuing education courses, academic courses, journals, and publications that relate to one's area of practice.	Ability to use resources such as newsletters, journals, and professional discussion groups to keep knowledgeable of trends. Ability to enroll in appropriate classes; ability to read appropriate publications.

Nursing Activities

Nursing activities related to continuing education are nurse-directed, rather than client-directed. The behaviors expected are that the holistic nurse seek out new knowledge in generalist nursing practice (for example, knowledge related to issues and trends in the discipline); new knowledge in the specific area in which the nurse is employed (for example, the nurse practicing in home care would be expected to seek out specific knowledge related to home care practice); and new knowledge in the field of holistic nursing (for example, knowledge related to development and testing of holistic nursing theory or knowledge related to understanding effects of holistic modalities).

CASE STUDIES

1 Nurse Cheryl was practicing in home care through a visiting nurses' association. Her practice was based at a neighborhood center, and one of her client groups was home-bound elderly living in an urban area. Cheryl maintained her currency in practice over the past two years by attending a conference for home care nurses that focused on how to obtain data from a community assessment of client needs; completing a home-study continuing education course on risk factors for injury for frail elderly; and completing a multidisciplinary workshop on the use of groupwork and reminiscence in car-

ing for elderly. Cheryl discussed her approaches to clients with other nurses with whom she works, and the nurses in her work setting have monthly meetings where the nurse manager informs Cheryl and the others about the trends related to organization and reimbursement of nursing services. In addition, Cheryl maintained membership in two nursing organizations and received and reviewed newsletters and published information from each of them.

Cheryl's work is in compliance with Standard 1.2.1. She is actively involved with the discipline of nursing and keeps herself informed of nursing activities related to her client population. Further, she explores holistic modalities (groupwork and reminiscence) as appropriate to her practice.

2 Nurse Maredean practiced in a birthing center for several years. She attended hour-long monthly continuing education meetings sponsored by the center. These meetings focused on the issues of providing safe and up-to-date care to women giving birth. She received continuing education credits for attending these meetings, as required by her state to renew her nursing license. She did not belong to any nursing organization, nor did she read any nursing publication (newsletter, newspaper, or journal) on a regular basis.

Maredean's continuing educational efforts are in keeping with her state law regarding currency of practice—she obtained the credits necessary for relicensure—but her efforts are not in keeping with Standard 1.2.1 for holistic nurses because she is not initiating her own continuing education efforts. She is not establishing a continuing education plan, nor is she reading the basic information on trends in her area of practice.

Standard of Practice 1.2.2

Holistic nurses identify areas of knowledge from nursing and various fields such as biomedicine, epidemiology, behavioral medicine, and cultural and social theories.

A holistic nurse understands that many disciplines and fields of study provide a basis for nursing practice. Recognizing that the client is a whole being with body-mind-spirit interconnectedness, the holistic nurse must have background in basic and advanced nursing knowledge and related fields to understand the client and to provide individualized care. Table 1–8 summarizes Standard 1.2.2.

Table 1–8 Harmony, Unity, and Healing in the Nursing Profession

Standard of Practice 1.2.2	*Key Concepts*	*Requisite Knowledge*	*Requisite Skills*
Holistic nurses identify areas of knowledge from nursing and various field such as biomedicine,	Nursing knowledge. Related fields: biomedicine, epidemiology,	Knowledge of nursing and holistic nursing practice beyond the basic level required for licensure.	Ability to attend continuing education programs and continue learning about nursing.

continues

Table 1–8 continued

Standard of Practice 1.2.2	*Key Concepts*	*Requisite Knowledge*	*Requisite Skills*
epidemiology, behavioral medicine, and social and cultural theories.	behavioral medicine, social/cultural theories.	Knowledge of related disciplines that directly apply to the nurse's practice area.	Ability to attend academic classes, sessions, or workshops that provide updates on disciplines related to nursing practice.

Nursing Activities

Holistic nurses keep up with nursing and related fields in many ways. These include attending continuing education courses, reading professional journals, reading review journals and review articles to learn of new developments in other fields, and attending university classes. Holistic nurses read in areas beyond their immediate scope of practice. For example, a pediatric nurse will keep up with knowledge of pediatrics and also with theories of culture particularly as related to parenting practices; a critical care nurse will attend classes to learn of new developments in biomedical practices. All holistic nurses will seek out epidemiological information on the health status of persons in their own communities. Thus, a basic understanding of fields other than nursing is required for holistic practice, and the ability to keep up with new developments and new findings in fields related to nursing is a part of the holistic nurse's professional practice.

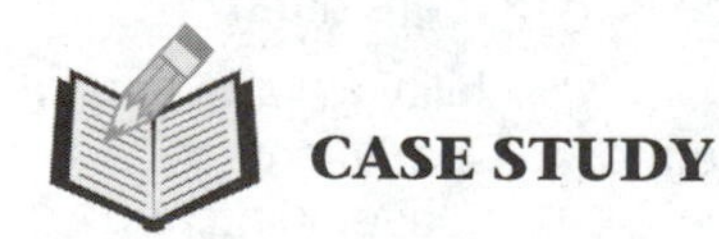

CASE STUDY

1 Jane was a parish nurse in a congregation close to the downtown area of a large city. There were many Hispanic families in the parish. Jane knew that the incidence of diabetes was high in the population she served, and she kept up with new developments in diabetic care through reading and attending workshops sponsored annually by the American Diabetic Association. She also attended a series of continuing education courses on Transcultural Care. Jane was interested in developing skills in transcultural communication. She learned of a class taught by an anthropology professor on the Hispanic Culture in America and signed up for the class.

Jane seeks out knowledge that will help to make her care culturally competent as well as current in her field. She has adopted a commitment to lifelong learning and will continue to develop her ability to provide quality care. Her actions are in keeping with Standard 1.2.2.

Standard of Practice 1.2.3

Holistic nurses continually develop and standardize holistic nursing guidelines, protocols, and practice to promote competency in holistic nursing practice and ensure quality of care to individuals.

Standard of Practice 1.2.4

Holistic nurses use the results of quality care activities to initiate change in holistic nursing practice.

Taken together, these two Standards deal with the need for evaluation of outcomes of nursing care to monitor quality. Knowing how and under what conditions quality care can be achieved, the nurse is called upon to develop new standards, revise existing standards, and/or write protocols to promote quality practices. Information published in the literature, as well as personal evaluation of outcomes, is used to establish levels of competency. Table 1–9 summarizes Standards 1.2.3 and 1.2.4.

Table 1–9 Development of Standards

Standards of Practice 1.2.3 and 1.2.4	*Key Concepts*	*Requisite Knowledge*	*Requisite Skills*
Holistic nurses continually develop and standardize holistic nursing guidelines, protocols, and practice to promote competency in holistic nursing practice and ensure quality of care to individuals, and use the results of quality care activities to initiate change in holistic nursing practice.	Develop and standardize guidelines for practice. Promote competency through written statements. Use quality care activities to initiate change.	Evaluations of outcomes of nursing practice. Knowledge of published literature.	Ability to read and understand quality care data. Ability to write and to participate in developing and revising standards and/or protocols for practice.

Nursing Activities

Activities that demonstrate meeting this Standard include: reviewing current literature to understand when there is need to change practice; volunteering to serve on committees that develop protocols and policies/procedures; working within AHNA and other nursing organizations to develop Standards of Practice; and participating in quality assurance activities to evaluate the outcome of nursing interventions.

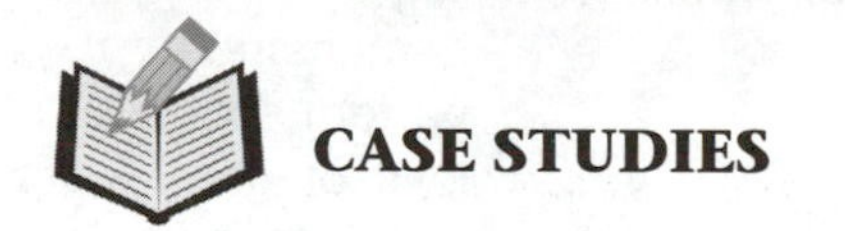

CASE STUDIES

1 Carol worked in a major medical center as a nurse researcher. She conducted a study on depression, social supports, and quality of life in older adults with osteoarthritis.[7] Her study results indicated that informal social supports play an important role in moderating the effects of the disease. Nurse Lorraine used the findings of Carol's study to evaluate practices at her center's outpatient clinic. She assessed the social supports available to the client population and the nurses' awareness of their patients' home situations. She worked with two other nurses to rewrite a nursing health history tool used at the clinic so that the tool included questions related to perceived social supports, attachment, problem solving, and self-management skills. Thus, Lorraine initiated changes in protocols of practice to incorporate new findings.

Lorraine's efforts help to ensure that all clients receive more comprehensive care. Her actions are in keeping with Standards 1.2.3 and 1.2.4 because she used her knowledge to develop guidelines for practice and thereby initiated positive changes in practice.

2 Ivan is a holistic nurse and had been a member of AHNA for several years. He came home from work one day to find a survey in the mail from AHNA national office. The survey asked him to complete information related to his practice as part of a revision of the Standards of Holistic Nursing Practice. Ivan read through the 11-page survey and realized that it would take him about one hour to complete the survey responsibly. He allowed time the following night to sit quietly and complete the survey, providing all the information he could.

Ivan's actions are in keeping with Standard 1.2.3 because he assisted in the process of developing and revising the Standards of Practice by providing accurate and reliable feedback to the ongoing process.

Standard of Practice 1.2.5

Holistic nurses may seek certification in holistic nursing as one means of advancing the philosophy and practice of holistic nursing.

Nurses seek certification to make a public statement about the value of studying, reflecting, and practicing holistic nursing. The certification process advances the philosophy and practice of holistic nursing by drawing attention to the fact that holistic nursing is a specialty and that there is a body of knowledge and an art of practice associated with the specialty. Holistic nurses are encouraged to seek certification and then to use the letters "HNC" to identify the specialty. Table 1–10 summarizes Standard 1.2.5.

Table 1–10 Certification

Standard of Practice 1.2.5	*Key Concepts*	*Requisite Knowledge*	*Requisite Skills*
Holistic nurses may seek certification in holistic nursing as one means of advancing the philosophy and practice of holistic nursing.	Seek certification. Advancing the philosophy and practice of holistic nursing.	Standards of Practice.	Ability to demonstrate performance at level of competency. Willingness to make a public statement about the practice of the specialty.

Nursing Activities

Activities that support this Standard include taking continuing education courses in holistic nursing, attending university classes in holistic nursing and related fields, completing a fieldwork practicum, seeking a mentor with whom to work, and completing the required portfolio and examination to demonstrate competency through the certification process. Further, study from the *AHNA Core Curriculum for Holistic Nursing*[8] supports this Standard, as the published Core Curriculum presents the foundation for the certification process.

CASE STUDY

1 Vita took a series of continuing education courses in holistic nursing. After three years' time, she saw herself as knowledgeable at a fairly advanced level. She then decided to enroll in a certificate program in holistic nursing so that she could develop her skills with the help of a mentor. She particularly wanted to apply holistic nursing theory to her practice and felt a mentor could guide her through this new process.

Having completed the certificate program, Vita decided to apply for certification in holistic nursing. She was studying for the examination when her friends from work called her and asked her to go to a movie. She declined, saying she was preparing for a certification exam. Her friends asked: "Why? You have a certificate, why do you need more? What does the certification mean to you?"

Vita thought for a moment or two and then replied: "I am committed to this process because a public statement about my knowledge and skill in holistic nursing is important to me. I want to be able to write 'HNC' after my name and let others know that there are many of us with this specialty of practice."

Vita's actions and commitment are in keeping with Standard 1.2.5. She is seeking out formal certification to document her own knowledge and skill and declares that there is a benefit to letting others know that there are many holistic nurses who claim a specialty in practice.

CONCLUSION

Core Value 1 provides the basis for all of holistic nursing practice. The philosophy of holism is a statement of values and beliefs that form the foundation of nurse relationships with others and with the environment. Holistic philosophy is the search for meaning, the perspective that values all life, and a belief in the interconnectedness of the body-mind-spirit. The basis of holistic education is that the nurse will commit to lifelong learning. Holistic nurses live professional and personal lives that expand their knowledge and understanding of human beings, of nursing, and of themselves. Core Value 1 is a prerequisite to the other Core Values, as the Standards described permeate all practice—and, indeed, the lives—of holistic nurses.

NOTES

1. *Oxford English Dictionary*, "Philosophy" (New York: Oxford University Press, 1971), 781.
2. S. Gortner, "Nursing Values and Science: Toward a Science Philosophy," in *Perspectives on Nursing Theory*, 3d ed., ed. L.H. Nicoll (Philadelphia: J.B. Lippincott Co., 1997), 197–206.
3. M. McKivergin, "The Nurse as an Instrument of Healing," in *Holistic Nursing: A Handbook for Practice*, 3d ed., eds. B. Dossey et al. (Gaithersburg, MD: Aspen Publishers, 2000), 207–212.
4. J. George and L. Frisch, "Theory and Neuroscience as a Basis for Practice," in *Psychiatric Mental Health Nursing: Understanding the Client as Well as the Condition*, eds. N. Frisch and L. Frisch (Albany, NY: Delmar Publishers, 1998), 27–67.
5. J. McCloskey and G. Bulechek, eds., "Hope Instillation," *Nursing Interventions Classification*, 2d ed. (St. Louis: Mosby, 1996), 321.
6. American Holistic Nurses' Association, *Code of Ethics for Holistic Nursing Practice* (Flagstaff, AZ: AHNA, 1992).
7. C. Blixen and C. Kippes, "Depression, Social Support, and Quality of Life in Older Adults with Osteoarthritis," *Image: The Journal of Nursing Scholarship* 31 (1999): 221–226.
8. B. Dossey, ed., *American Holistic Nurses' Association Core Curriculum for Holistic Nursing* (Gaithersburg, MD: Aspen Publishers, 1997).

CORE VALUE 2

HOLISTIC ETHICS, THEORIES, AND RESEARCH

Noreen Cavan Frisch

2.1 Holistic Ethics

■■ Holistic nurses hold to a professional ethic of caring and healing that seeks to preserve wholeness and dignity of self, students, colleagues, and the person who is receiving care in all practice settings, be it in health promotion, birthing centers, acute or chronic care facilities, end-of-life centers, or in homes. ■■

While ethics of practice are integral to all professional nursing, holistic nurses focus on their responsibility to provide care that maintains the human dignity of every person. The Ethics of Caring have been described well by nurse theorist Jean Watson and others who point out that care cannot be moral if a client, nurse, or other person involved in the client's care is treated as an object.[1] The nurse-client, nurse-nurse, and nurse-other relationships must be maintained within the context of human-to-human interaction. In addition, holistic nursing ethics include responsibilities that a nurse has to self, the client, coworkers, and the profession. The American Holistic Nurses' Association (AHNA) has developed a Code of Ethics,[2] presented in Exhibit 2–1. All care is grounded in this code. There are five Standards that relate to holistic ethics; each is discussed in the section following the presentation of the Code of Ethics.

Standard of Practice 2.1.1

Holistic nurses identify the ethics of caring and its contribution to unity of self, others, nature, and God/Life Force/Absolute/Transcendent as central to holistic nursing practice.

This Standard emphasizes the importance of the caring relationship and its impact on the sense of unity. The caring relationship is one built upon the need for true connection between and among human beings. The use of the word *caring* acknowledges that something or someone outside the person matters and creates personal concerns.[3] Caring sets up the condition where help can be given and received. The sense of unity is part of the harmony that comes with knowing one has connections with others, nature, and God/Life Force/Absolute/Transcendent. The ethics of caring contribute to the unfolding mystery of the spirit and, thus, are required for care to be considered whole. Table 2–1 illustrates Standard 2.1.1.

Exhibit 2–1 American Holistic Nurses' Association Code of Ethics

We believe that the fundamental responsibilities of the nurse are to promote health, facilitate healing, and alleviate suffering. The need for nursing is universal. Inherent in nursing is the respect for life, dignity, and rights of all persons. Nursing care is given in a context mindful of the holistic nature of humans, understanding the body-mind-spirit connection. Nursing care is unrestricted by considerations of nationality, race, creed, color, age, sex, sexual preference, politics, or social status. Given that nurses practice in culturally diverse settings, professional nurses must have an understanding of the cultural background of clients in order to provide culturally appropriate interventions.

Nurses render services to clients who can be individuals, families, groups, or communities. The client is an active participant in health care and should be included in all nursing care planning decisions.

In order to provide services to others, each nurse has a responsibility toward him/herself. In addition, nurses have defined responsibilities toward the client, co-workers, nursing practice, the profession of nursing, society, and the environment.

NURSES AND SELF

The nurse has a responsibility to model health behaviors. Holistic nurses strive to achieve harmony in their own lives and assist others striving to do the same.

NURSES AND THE CLIENT

The nurse's primary responsibility is to the client needing nursing care. The nurse strives to see the client as a whole and provides care that is professionally appropriate and culturally consonant. The nurse holds in confidence all information obtained in professional practice and uses professional judgment in disclosing such information. The nurse enters into a relationship with the client that is guided by mutual respect and a desire for growth and development.

NURSES AND CO-WORKERS

The nurse maintains cooperative relationships with co-workers in nursing and other fields. Nurses have a responsibility to nurture each other and to assist nurses to work as a team in the interest of client care. If a client's care is endangered by a co-worker, the nurse must take appropriate action on behalf of the client.

NURSES AND NURSING PRACTICE

The nurse carries personal responsibilities for practice and for maintaining continued competence. Nurses have the right to utilize all appropriate nursing interventions, and have the obligation to determine the efficacy and safety of all nursing actions. Wherever applicable, nurses utilize research findings in directing practice.

continues

Exhibit 2–1 continued

NURSES AND THE PROFESSION

The nurse plays a role in determining and implementing desirable standards of nursing practice and education. Holistic nurses may assume a leadership position to guide the profession toward holism. Nurses support nursing research and the development of holistically oriented nursing theories. The nurse participates in establishing and maintaining equitable social and economic working conditions in nursing.

NURSES AND SOCIETY

The nurse, along with other citizens, has responsibility for initiating and supporting actions to meet the health and social needs of the public.

NURSES AND THE ENVIRONMENT

The nurse strives to manipulate the client's environment to become one of peace, harmony, and nurturance so that healing may take place. The nurse considers the health of the ecosystem in relation to the need for health, safety, and peace of all persons.

Table 2–1 Ethics of Caring

Standard of Practice 2.1.1	*Key Concepts*	*Requisite Knowledge*	*Requisite Skills*
Holistic nurses identify the ethics of caring and its contribution to unity of self, others, nature, and God/Life Force/Absolute/Transcendent as central to holistic nursing practice.	Ethics of caring.	Ethical theories of care.	Ability to form relationships with clients.
	Unity of self, others, nature, and God/Life Force/Absolute/Transcendent.	Caring principles of trust, presence, empathy, concern.	Observational and assessment skills related to trust, vulnerability, and the personal meaning of lived experiences.

Nursing Activities

Nursing activities that demonstrate this Standard begin with accepting the sense that all practice, all techniques, and all nursing interventions are done within the context of a human-to-human interaction. The presence and thought of the holistic nurse underpins all assessments, analyses, actions, and work. Thus, the nurse's understanding that "caring" forms a framework within which all nursing takes place is the first step in meeting this Standard in practice. Secondly, this Standard requires that the nurse be open to relationships with clients—relationships that may leave the nurse as well as the client changed because of the significance of the interactions between the two. Benner points out that the "privileged place of nursing" puts nurses in touch with people in the midst of health, pain, loss, suffering, birth, and death.[3] To ethically accept this privileged place, nurses must accept relationships, must care about others, must recognize that caring puts them in a place of front-line intimacy, and go on to conduct nursing's work in the context of how each event is understood and experienced by the client. All nursing activities must be carried out with the intent to help, to support, to care, and to improve the health, coping, recovery, and sense of peace for the client. The client's sense of unity, harmony, peace, and hope are the means by which the nurse can evaluate his or her actions in relation to this Standard.

CASE STUDY

1 Cathy was working in a drug treatment center for adolescents. Her clients were high-school-aged students who had been involved with street drugs, alcohol abuse, and truancy. Her job was to support the interventions of a multidisciplinary treatment team and to provide group counseling, health assessments, and health education to the clients. She was working with Svetlana, a 16-year-old girl who had been brought to the center by her very concerned, and very distressed, parents. Svetlana had been a good student in school, but her grades started dropping. She admitted to use of marijuana, alcohol, and cocaine, and to having recently experimented with heroin. Svetlana entered into the center's group sessions for girls her age. She started drug counseling and signed a contract to attend sessions, return to school, and abstain from drugs. Based on the stress of Svetlana's relationship with her parents, she requested that she live at the center's group home for the time being. This request was granted, and she then had to agree to "house rules," including participating in house activities and chores, accepting a curfew, and maintaining a drug-free house. Cathy counseled her about the meaning of the contract she signed and the meaning of Svetlana's acceptance of the house rules. Cathy told her: "The center is able to provide treatment only to a few people. Those who are receiving our care must go along with the program—the full program of school, counseling, group, and rules. We can give you all we have, and our clients have had great success in finding lives without drugs, but you must know that clients must leave if our house rules are broken. Further, our program will provide you with ongoing help as long as you need it, provided that you work with the treatment plan."

The center was one that offered a program based on support, confrontation of reality, tough love, and absolute adherence to responsibility for consequences of one's actions. Cathy's actions and words, in and of themselves, do not demonstrate either meeting or not meeting this Standard. Cathy will meet this Standard if she enters into a caring relationship with Svetlana. Cathy does meet this Standard: Cathy has the perspective that Svetlana is a unique and wonderful human being, with great potential to develop into adulthood without addiction to drugs. Cathy understands that drug abuse is widespread and enticing, and that successful treatment recognizes the reasons for the abuse while making no excuses for the individual's behavior. Cathy tells Svetlana she will "be there for you" during the treatment. Cathy maintains her part of the contract—she will be where she says she will be; she cares for Svetlana and demonstrates this by assisting her to look at her life, providing help for her to cope, to recover, to build new relationships, and to heal her relationship with her parents. Cathy, however, is straightforward and truthful and does not accept excuses and manipulations. She recognizes that structure within the relationship and demand for honesty are part of the principle of caring. Cathy demonstrates in her relationship with Svetlana that caring for self is one of the first steps to recovery. Cathy knows that her recovery must include building a trusting relationship with another human being, so she offers herself as a trustworthy person.

It is the context of the care, the words, and the nurse-client relationship that demonstrate meeting Standard 2.1.1. It would be possible for a nurse to say all of the same things Cathy says and not meet the Standard, if that nurse did not accept and value the client, and did not think about Svetlana in the context of an individual who was unique and desperately needed to be cared for to bring about successful recovery.

Standard of Practice 2.1.2

Holistic nurses integrate the standards of holistic nursing practice with applicable state laws and regulations governing nursing practice.

It may go without saying that holistic nurses keep their work within the laws, regulations, and standards adopted by the states in which they are licensed. However, the practice of holistic nursing leaves some areas of practice ill-defined, and the nurse, to practice ethically and professionally, must have knowledge of those areas and a clear understanding of the meaning of state regulatory bodies. It is completely legal to practice holistically within every state of the United States. There are, however, restrictions on the practice of certain modalities in some locations. Further, the titles of nurses (for example, advanced-practice nurse, certified nurse, clinical nurse specialist, or nurse specialist) are titles protected by law in some states. Every nurse must know under what conditions a nurse may use these titles within his or her state. Table 2–2 provides a summary of Standard 2.1.2.

Table 2–2 Integration of Standards with State Laws/Regulations

Standard of Practice 2.1.2	*Key Concepts*	*Requisite Knowledge*	*Requisite Skills*
Holistic nurses integrate the standards of holistic nursing	Standards of holistic nursing practice.	Understanding of the standards.	Ability to apply the standards.

continues

Table 2–2 continued

Standard of Practice 2.1.2	*Key Concepts*	*Requisite Knowledge*	*Requisite Skills*
practice with applicable state laws and regulations governing nursing practice.	State laws and regulations.	Knowledge of the Nurse Practice Act in one's home state. Understanding of nursing's scope of practice. Knowledge of the regulations on practice.	Ability to interpret (or to obtain expert help in interpreting) the laws, scope of practice, and meanings of regulations on practice.

Nursing Activities

Holistic nurses must have a copy of the Nurse Practice Act regulating their work, and must keep informed of changes in law and regulations that could impact on the legal basis of their care. Holistic nurses always maintain legal practice and at times have taken leadership roles in seeking clarification and change in laws. Most states are governed by a Board of Nursing.* Members of State Boards of Nursing are usually appointed to those positions and meet specified requirements for education and practice.[4] Many states have nurses on their boards who represent nursing practice, nursing education, and nursing administration. Some states also require that a public member who is not a nurse serve on the State Board. The laws that dictate nursing practice are written at the state level, and practice laws differ somewhat across state lines. State Boards of Nursing in most states are responsible for interpreting the state law for nurses through the statement of regulations dictating very specific areas of practice. Particularly in relation to holistic nurses, questions relating to modalities (such as "May a Registered Nurse practice massage therapy?") are directed to and answered by the State Board of Nursing. Holistic nurses must be aware of the fact that not all State Boards will answer such questions in the same way.

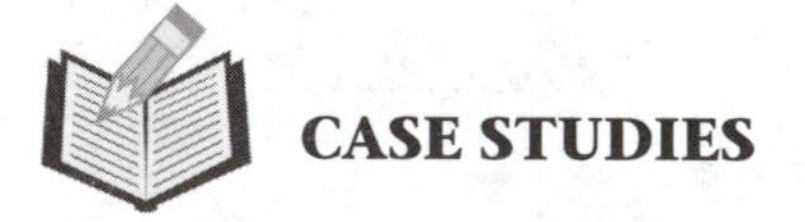

CASE STUDIES

1 Nurse Tom was completing a continuing education program in guided imagery. He was a Master's prepared nurse with a practice specialty in rehabilitation nursing. He worked at a rehabilitation hospital with clients who had

*In states such as Illinois where there is no State Board of Nursing, there is a regulatory body that governs the practice of licensed professionals. Nurses must know the particular situation in their own state.

suffered multiple injuries. He took the guided imagery program because he thought the modality would help him to assist his clients, who are in pain, who have lost muscle function, and who deal daily with high levels of stress. Tom inquired of his agency and his State Board of Nursing regarding the practice of guided imagery in his work. His board of nursing defined guided imagery as within the scope of practice for an RN who can demonstrate expertise in the modality. His employer—the institution—was very interested in his new skill. His supervisor stated that they had no written policies, procedures, or guidelines governing the practice within the institution. At the supervisor's request, Tom wrote a draft of these and, in time, the institution accepted a written policy regarding nurses' use of guided imagery in practice. Tom did not incorporate guided imagery into his care until he knew that the practice was legal in his state and until his employer had guidelines governing its use within the institution.

Tom's practice is in keeping with Standard 2.1.2, as he is integrating the modality of guided imagery into his care, but doing so only after careful review of his state's laws. Further, he is instrumental in developing guidelines for the use of guided imagery at his institution. He is keeping his holistic nursing practice within the laws of his state and the regulations of his employer.

2 Nurse Susan was a nurse massage-therapist who had been an advocate for the practice of massage in nursing for many years. She took on a leadership role in the area by becoming a liaison for nurses in two national organizations defining the practice of massage and touch within nursing. She submitted definitions of touch, simple touch, therapeutic use of touch, simple massage, and massage therapy to her State Board of Nursing for consideration. Through a very lengthy process of education, documentation, research, and advocacy, Susan was instrumental in having her State Board adopt definitions of these therapies so that they could become incorporated into nursing practice in her state. Susan kept her practice within the legal scope defined in her state and then advocated for the adoption of new regulations.

Susan's efforts not only meet Standard 2.1.2, but they exceed the Standard by helping to move holistic nursing forward.

3 Nurse Velma completed a course in hypnotherapy in the state adjacent to where she lives. She worked in geriatric care, and her practice was based at an adult day health center. She began to apply what she learned in her work. She made no effort to inquire about the practice of hypnotherapy in her state.

Velma's actions are not in keeping with Standard 2.1.2 and may be illegal in her state. She should determine the legal basis for the practice of hypnotherapy in the state where she is practicing before she implements the modality.

Standard of Practice 2.1.3

Holistic nurses engage in activities that respect, nurture, and enhance the integral relationship with the earth, and advocate for the well-being of the global community's economy, education, and social justice.

This Standard calls on the nurse to extend his or her thoughts outside the immediate world of a practice setting and home environment. The health of the planet, as well as the needs of persons globally, affects all. Holistic nurses think in terms of the whole and in terms of relationships with others. Social and environmental justice are necessary to heal the world and to bring peace and harmony to the world. The AHNA Position Statement in Support of a Healthful Environment[5] and Position Statement on Social Issues[6] help to illustrate the meaning of this Standard. These are presented in Exhibits 2–2 and 2–3.

Exhibit 2–2 The AHNA Position Statement in Support of a Healthful Environment

The philosophy of the AHNA includes the belief that "health involves the harmonious balance of body, mind, and spirit in an ever-changing environment."

The environment involves our immediate, as well as global, surroundings. Many of us are aware of a need to expand our consciousness regarding environmental issues and believe that this can have an effect on our own person and community well-being.

Our concern comes from a reverence for the beauty and integrity of the earth that sustains us and is our home, our Mother Earth. Relevant environmental issues include preserving the integrity of the air, soil, and water as well as issues such as global warming, acid rain, and other equally challenging situations. We believe, as holistic nurses, that we have a responsibility for increasing awareness regarding these issues in others, through role modeling and educating within our communities.

The AHNA encourages self-responsible behavior as well as participation in socially responsible environmental groups, to protect and support improvement of the health of our environment.

Exhibit 2–3 The AHNA Position Statement on Social Issues

The philosophy of the AHNA includes the belief that "health involves the harmonious balance of body, mind, and spirit in an ever-changing environment."

Thus, every individual can be viewed as having three components—body, mind, and spirit—that interconnect in making the whole. Harmonious balance is achieved when conditions in an individual's life support and enhance the growth and development of each component.

Modern life presents threats and/or challenges to an individual's wholeness whenever necessary supports for physical safety, environmen-

continues

Exhibit 2–3 continued

tal health, cognitive growth, and spiritual development are not present. AHNA supports promotion of conditions in society and in the world community that contribute to achieving universal opportunity for full development of every person. We recognize that many of these conditions are controlled by public policy and governmental decisions. For this reason, the association strives to keep its members informed of relevant social concerns and political decisions so that members may influence policy whenever possible to achieve equality and justice for all persons.

AHNA encourages socially responsible behaviors of its members regarding the nursing profession and the health care system and encourages advocacy for those groups in need of support to achieve conditions necessary for holism.

Table 2–3 summarizes Standard 2.1.3.

Table 2–3 Relationship with the Earth

Standard of Practice 2.1.3	*Key Concepts*	*Requisite Knowledge*	*Requisite Skills*
Holistic nurses engage in activities that respect, nurture, and enhance the integral relationship with the earth, and advocate for the well-being of the global community's economy, education, and social justice.	Relationship of humans to the earth. Well-being of the global community's economy, education, and social justice.	Environmental health issues. Economic, educational, political, and social activities, and their relationships to health.	Analysis of environmental and population data. Social/political advocacy. Public education.

Nursing Activities

Nursing activities that demonstrate meeting this Standard include: analysis of community and population data to determine the level of health and level of health risk faced by a community; public education efforts regarding environmental health; analysis and evaluation of social conditions in a community that foster health, growth, and well-being; and public advocacy aimed at increasing social justice.

While every holistic nurse may not be an expert in the field of environmental health, it is assumed that every holistic nurse understands the interconnectedness of humans and the earth—i.e., that the health of the planet is necessary for the health of humankind. Awareness of factors that deplete the environment—pollution, hazardous waste, hazardous emissions, and destruction of habitat—call upon every holistic nurse to examine his or her own life patterns and to make changes in the service of each person's contribution to global health. Nurses who may not have the skills to assess environmental health hazards or risks are expected to consult with environmental experts in their community or to read and assess the published work on the topic to fully understand the factors relevant to themselves and their clients.

Issues of social justice that bear upon the health of the community are equally as important as those related to the environment. Holistic nurses should assess topics of greatest concern to their own community and/or own clients. Factors such as violence, suicide, alcohol and/or drug addiction, and unwanted pregnancies are examples of social problems that affect the health of all. Nurses should be aware not only of the problems but also of the proposed solutions in their localities. When the timing is appropriate, the holistic nurse can advocate for social policies that impact on community well-being.

CASE STUDIES

1 Marita was a pediatric nurse living in a rural community in the Northwest. The town in which she lived had a population of about 10,000 people. The town was located near a river that had been fished for salmon and used for recreational swimming, canoeing, etc. Members of her community learned that the number of fish was declining and that industrial and logging activities upstream were causing changes in the river. Biologists conducted evaluations of the area and determined that the health of the river was dependent upon changes in industry. Marita could see that there was a problem that seemed unfixable as people from the "industry" and from the "environmental" sides of the problem were making demands on one another. She realized that the decision of what to do to "save the river" and "save the community" would be made politically. She sought to inform herself of the issues through reading and discussions with involved parties. She talked to members of her town council. Some of the concerns Marita had, as a citizen and as a pediatric nurse, were issues of community life and recreational opportunities for children, and whether the river could be preserved for these activities. She also informed herself of the projected economic impact of changes in employment on her client families. She then sought to support community actions that would inform community members of the facts involved. It became apparent to Marita that many persons were speaking about this issue without complete knowledge of the problem and were making judgments based on no data. Marita knew that restrictions on industry could result from political and legal efforts, that there were people who were truly looking for a solution that could meet at least some of the community's economic needs, understanding that the

health of the river would be a measure of the health of the ecosystem. Marita directed her community volunteer efforts at public education and understanding, which she believed to be a precursor to sound decision making.

Marita's actions as a citizen and as a nurse are in keeping with Standard 2.1.3. She is taking the situation seriously, attempting to gain knowledge, and assisting those in the community to obtain information. She consults with experts in the subject—she does not assume that one side of the issue is always "right" and one is not. Her actions are in keeping with the need of holistic nurses to maintain knowledge and work within their communities.

2 Jorge was a big-city person. He was a nurse in an intensive care unit at a large urban medical center. He lived in a suburb with his family. He drove 40 miles to work every day (one way), his wife drove 45 miles to work—each commuted in the same direction but at slightly different times. His car was a large, four-wheel-drive sport utility vehicle that he took onto the freeway. When he purchased the SUV, he thought that he would be driving out to the country for hiking and outdoor activities, but he really never had much time for that. He was a busy person, moving well along a professional career path. Frequently, he would not get home for dinner until quite late because he served on several hospital committees. He ate fast food; he bought his morning café latte at a stand where he drank out of a disposable paper cup. His wife was equally busy—though she usually got home before he did to relieve the babysitter in the late afternoon. They had two children, one still in diapers (disposable, due to lack of time to wash diapers). They haven't worked recycling into their family patterns, even though curbside recycling is available in their suburb—they are simply too busy. They took pride in their new, 4,000-square-foot home and its two acres of land with beautiful green lawn. Recently they received a flyer in their mailbox from a person selling a new technique to water lawns with a gray-water recycling system. Jorge couldn't understand what the flyer was all about. He said, "Why would anybody do that? We have plenty of water in our sprinkling system as it is!"

Jorge has adopted the enticing lifestyle of American affluence. Concerns for the environment have escaped his consciousness. He is not acting in keeping with Standard 2.1.3.

Standard of Practice 2.1.4

Holistic nurses advocate for the rights of patients to have educated choices into their plan of care.

This Standard is based on the principle of "autonomy," the ethical principle regarding the individual's right to self-determination and independence.[7] The principle of autonomy is understood in relation to the client's right to informed consent. Clients have the right to be given clear information about treatment options, risks, benefits, and alternatives. To give consent for treatment, an individual must be alert and oriented, must understand the procedure or treatment being offered, and must freely (without coercion) accept the treatment. Further, clients have the right to refuse treatment, to consent to treatment while refusing specific treatments, and, where consent has been given, to withdraw consent at any time. Table 2–4 summarizes this Standard.

Table 2–4 Autonomy

Standard of Practice 2.1.4	*Key Concepts*	*Requisite Knowledge*	*Requisite Skills*
Holistic nurses advocate for the rights of patients to have educated choices into their plan of care.	Autonomy. Informed consent.	Laws regarding informed consent. The Principle of Autonomy. Knowledge of treatment choices suggested in specific cases.	Client education skills. Analytical skills regarding treatment choices.

Nursing Activities

The nursing activities in keeping with this Standard include, first and foremost, commitment to the client's right to choose treatment. Second, the nurse must have current knowledge of the laws within his or her state that define the requirements for informed consent and those conditions (e.g., emergencies, care of minors, care of specified psychiatric conditions) where informed consent can be waived. With this knowledge, the holistic nurse may be involved in client education programs, discussions with clients about their choices, and the provision of information on subjects such as "advance directives" and "living wills." Often, holistic nurses are questioned by clients about topics and treatment choices for which there is little research data or published information on efficacy. The nurse must provide information that is credible on all complementary or alternative modalities or provide a referral or references to the best source of knowledge. Holistic nurses are aware of the fact that there are few research data on many of the modalities the public would like to know about. Nurses must take care not to represent a treatment as helpful without data documenting that this is so. The National Center for Complementary and Alternative Medicine at the National Institutes of Health is a national clearinghouse for public, as well as professional, information on such modalities. The nurse may access its Web site at http://www.nccam.nih.gov.

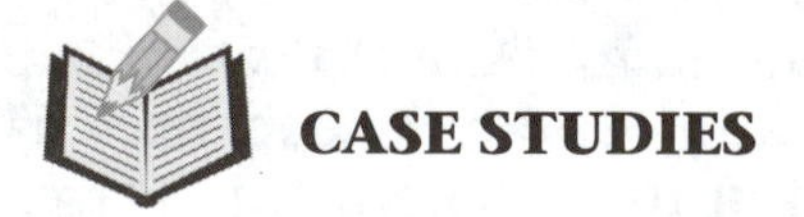

CASE STUDIES

1 Nurse Gloria worked in an oncology department of an ambulatory care clinic. She interacted daily with clients who had cancer diagnoses, assisting them primarily in scheduling outpatient chemotherapy treatments and arranging for referrals to home care nursing, as well as taking any measures she could to assist clients to follow their treatment plans. At times a client would ask her about complementary treatments to the recommended plan.

Gloria was a relatively new nurse to this discipline. She was learning about the standard, recommended conventional treatments offered. She was also learning about activities in her community that were supportive to clients with cancer. There were resources through the American Cancer Society, including some support groups. There were weekend workshops offered by cancer survivors to speak directly with clients and their families about the experience of illness. There was also a small group of holistic nurses who offered treatments in guided imagery and healing touch to clients. She learned from a parish nurse that there were local churches that offered intercessory prayer for members of their congregations and others who wished to be remembered in prayer. Gloria collected information about each of these activities and first made the information available to her colleagues at the clinic. She found that many of her colleagues were familiar with at least some of these services. She asked at a team meeting if information about these community groups could be made available to clients on a regular basis. It was decided by the group that the clinic would provide written information about these services on a table in the clinic to let clients know that these services were available.

Gloria then discovered that clients would ask her what she knew and what she thought about these services. Gloria took care to limit her answers to what was known about the modality or service in question. For example, Gloria told a woman with breast cancer who asked about a support group that "many women with breast cancer have found such groups helpful. In fact, while there are only a small number of research studies on the topic, those that have been done support the use of these groups." Then Gloria went on to ask the client about herself: "Have you been thinking about going to one of these groups?" to open up communication and to be supportive to her client's needs. In another case, a man undergoing treatment for Hodgkin's disease stated that he just couldn't stand the side effects, particularly the nausea, following treatments. He took the antiemetic drugs, but he asked: "Is there anything else I can do?" Gloria mentioned that there were some patients who find the use of imagery helpful. After brief discussion, Gloria referred him to the nurse providing the modality so that specific questions about the modality could be answered.

Gloria's actions are consistent with Standard 2.1.4. As a new nurse to the field of oncology, she is learning daily about the treatments, the clients, and the supports available in her community. She took action to help make information available to clients. She does not operate from an assumption that *every* client needs or wants all of the support services available. For example, she provided correct information about use of support groups for women with breast cancer but did not assume that her client would go to a support group. Rather, she asked her client what the client's own thoughts were about support groups to begin the process of helping the client consider alternatives and make the best choices about her own care.

2 Nurse Peggy worked in an acute surgical unit of a hospital. Most of the clients she saw were orthopaedic patients immediately post-op. She received Frank, a 25-year-old man, to her unit. Frank had been in a car accident that morning and suffered multiple injuries to his leg. He had surgery to insert a pin into the femur that would reduce the fractures and allow a cast to be applied. She assessed Frank's status upon his transfer from the Recovery Room: he was stable, experiencing pain, and asking for help. Peggy administered morphine as ordered for pain and assessed that the medication did reduce the pain. Knowing that comfort would be a high nursing priority for Frank, Peggy continued to monitor his level of discomfort and offered medications as ordered.

While Peggy is providing professionally responsible care, her care is not in keeping with this Standard. She correctly identified that control of pain is a nursing priority for Frank, and she provided medications accordingly. However, she made no effort to ascertain whether other comfort measures could be used, would be acceptable to Frank, and could, potentially, increase the effects Frank obtains from the medications. In keeping with this Standard, a holistic nurse would offer comfort measures that could include positioning, distractions, imagery, therapeutic touch (TT), and music therapy, among others. Only when a range of interventions is offered to clients do the clients have the ability to make informed choices about their treatment plans.

Standard of Practice 2.1.5

Holistic nurses participate in peer evaluation to ensure knowledge and competency in holistic nursing practice.

Holistic nurses participate in many forms of peer evaluation to ensure that their practice is appropriate. Attendance at continuing education offerings on the philosophy of holism, on the legal basis for practice, and on any of the modalities nurses may use all assist a nurse to maintain currency and compare his or her practice with those of others. College- or university-level courses in holism and holistic nursing offer an opportunity for a nurse to compare his or her ideas and practices against those of peers and experts in the field. And, of course, certificate programs and Master's degree programs offer nurses the opportunity to take courses and undergo an evaluation process to ensure that their practice meets with identified national standards. (A list of certificate programs endorsed by the AHNA and a list of Master's-level nursing programs offering emphasis on holistic nursing are included in Appendixes C and D.)

Additionally, in keeping with the intent of this Standard, holistic nurses who are experts in holism and in the practice of specific modalities are called upon to mentor, coach, and support nurses learning the practices. Further, nurses who are experts should participate in committees that develop and improve upon Standards of Practice, keeping the Standards current and relevant.

Table 2–5 presents a summary of Standard 2.1.5.

Table 2–5 Peer Evaluation

Standard of Practice 2.1.5	*Key Concepts*	*Requisite Knowledge*	*Requisite Skills*
Holistic nurses participate in peer evaluation to ensure knowledge and competency in holistic nursing practice.	Peer evaluation, peer review. Currency in knowledge and practice.	Knowledge of certificate and educational programs.	Willingness to learn, to share, and to have own work be reviewed by peers in the field.

Nursing Activities

Activities that demonstrate meeting this Standard are participation in certificate programs, Master's degree programs, and continuing education activities. Further, many of the activities sponsored by AHNA local networks—those that involve nursing rounds and presentations of case studies for discussion and review—demonstrate how nurses are meeting this Standard. Additionally, for many nurses, annual reviews by a superior in the work setting provide peer review and information with which to evaluate and improve one's own work.

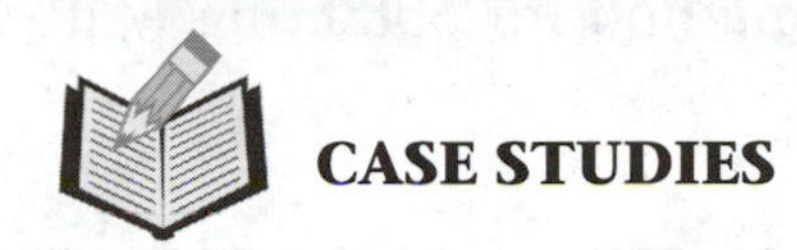

CASE STUDIES

1 Carolyn was preparing for certification in Holistic Nursing. She enrolled in a certificate program to prepare herself for the formal certification process. She had a small private practice in Healing Touch (in which she already carried certification as a practitioner), and worked for a home care agency providing home assessments and visits to clients. She selected cases from the home care practice for case studies in her certificate program and sought out a mentor (an expert holistic nurse who was on the faculty of a local university) to review and comment on her practice. Carolyn went through a process of obtaining review of her work for a period of one year before she presented herself for certification.

Her actions clearly demonstrate meeting Standard 2.1.5 because she actively sought out a mentoring relationship wherein she could receive expert feedback about her work.

2 Shawna, an expert nurse in physiological nursing, was a doctorally prepared nurse who had a faculty position at a university. Her practice was grounded in nursing theory and she was an expert in qualitative research. She was a holistic nurse by philosophy, committed to meeting the needs of the whole person. Shawna volunteered to bring a case study of a challenging client with whom she had worked to a local AHNA network meeting. She presented the case, described the challenges in meeting her client's needs, and asked for the group to think about approaches and techniques that might help in client care.

Shawna also is meeting this Standard, as she is actively seeking the input of other holistic nurses in thinking about how to give the best care to a challenging client.

Standard of Practice 2.1.6

Holistic nurses protect the personal privacy and confidentiality of individuals, especially with health care agencies and managed care organizations.

This Standard is based on the client's right to privacy. Privacy is the right of any client to keep personal information secret.[8] Thus, any client has the right to keep the fact that she is a client, that she is in treatment, or that she has a diagnosis to herself. There are times when a person may not want his or her spouse, employer, friends, or others to know that care is being received. In honoring that right, professional codes of behavior frequently state that confidentiality may not be breached. The AHNA Code of Ethics includes such a statement: "The nurse holds in confidence all information obtained in professional practice. . ."[2]

Holistic nurses, particularly those in private practice, may wish to file third-party claims to be reimbursed for their services. These nurses must be aware that when filing a claim to an insurer, the nurse is asked to provide information regarding the client's status, diagnosis, treatments, etc. Such claims cannot be filed without the informed consent of the client to disclose information to the insurer. A nurse with a private practice is advised to have in place a business plan that includes appropriate methods of payment for services and, if third-party reimbursement is planned, a clear method for obtaining written client permission.

Table 2–6 is a summary of Standard 2.1.6.

Table 2–6 Right to Privacy

Standard of Practice 2.1.6	*Key Concepts*	*Requisite Knowledge*	*Requisite Skills*
Holistic nurses protect the personal privacy and confidentiality of individuals, especially with health care agencies and managed care organizations.	Confidentiality. Protection of client's privacy.	Meaning of the "right to privacy." Laws governing disclosure of information.	Willingness to advocate for the client's rights.

Nursing Activities

Activities that demonstrate meeting this Standard include ensuring that any person involved in a case discussion about a client has a professional interest or "need to know" about the case; refraining from talking about clients in public places; keeping client records in appropriate files; and not disclosing confidential information over the telephone to an unseen caller. Further, the nurse must have a process in place to obtain clients' consent to discuss their case with others, including filing claims for third-party reimbursement.

There are specific situations, identified by law, where disclosure of client information is required—for example, cases where the client is potentially homicidal or suicidal, cases where the client is a minor, and cases where the client may be judged to be legally incompetent.[9] The nurse is advised to maintain current knowledge of such issues within his or her home state and/or to seek legal counsel if there is a question regarding the client's right to privacy and the nurse's legal obligation to share information.

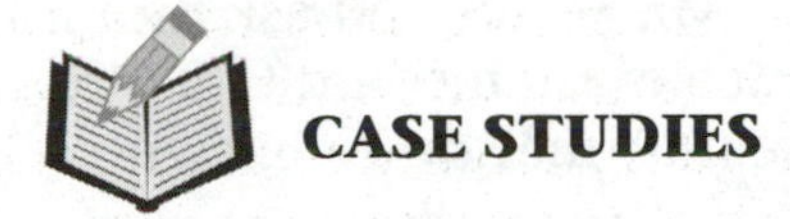

CASE STUDIES

1 Michelle was a nurse with a private practice in holistic nursing. She provided health education activities and stress reduction, and practiced the modalities of healing touch and guided imagery. She had an office in a suburb of a large city. She kept her own client records and had a secretary assist her with her front office, telephone, and billing. Mr. Kay, an executive from a nearby company, made an appointment to see Michelle for stress and lifestyle issues after he was screened for hypertension and found that his blood pressure was elevated. Mr. Kay was a bit nervous about seeing a holistic health provider, but he said he wanted to "keep all of my options open" and to "try out anything that may help." Upon the first visit, Mr. Kay stated he had health insurance but did not wish Michelle's secretary to bill the company since he was the owner of the business. Further, he wanted Michelle to keep confidential all visits and treatments discussed and offered. He asked that Michelle keep no records of his visits to her office. Michelle said that she was more than willing to keep in confidence the fact that he was a client of hers and said that her secretary also would keep in confidence the fact that he was a client. Further, Michelle stated that she would not have to bill insurance, as long as other arrangements could be made for payment. However, Michelle explained that she must keep professional records of office visits—she was in a professional practice. Mr. Kay maintained a right to review what was in the records, but the records must stay in her office, as all of the records of her clients were there. After a few minutes' discussion of the problem, Mr. Kay related that he was really worried that people who worked with him would think he was silly if they knew he was visiting a holistic healer. Michelle was able to honestly reassure him that she was a registered nurse, that her practice was based on nationally accepted standards of care, that she held certification in two modalities, and that she served many highly educated individuals. During this discussion Mr. Kay became more comfortable with the visit and gave Michelle permission to keep client records as she would for any client. Michelle again reassured Mr. Kay that all discussions were kept confidential. They agreed not to submit bills to Mr. Kay's insurance.

Michelle's practice is in keeping with this Standard. She maintains her client's right to privacy, and at the same time she maintains her own professional obligation to keep records of her practice.

2 Yuri was a nurse in a critical care unit. He received a phone call from a woman who stated that she was Mrs. Seeter, the wife of a man just admitted to the unit. Mrs. Seeter asked whether her husband was on the unit and what his status was. Yuri disclosed the requested information about his new patient but later worried whether he had done the right thing.

Yuri's actions are not in keeping with Standard 2.1.5. He is not legally able to disclose information about his clients to unknown persons over the telephone. Of course, Yuri wanted to help a family member in a situation of crisis. His best response might have been to go to the bedside of Mr. Seeter and ask him if he wanted to talk to the woman on the phone. Mr. Seeter then could talk directly to his spouse and give Yuri permission to disclose information to his wife.

2.2 Holistic Nursing Theories

■■ ***Holistic nurses recognize that holistic nursing theories provide the framework for all aspects of holistic nursing practice and transformational leadership.*** ■■

There are many theories that provide a framework for nursing care and practice. Some were developed within the profession of nursing; some were borrowed from other disciplines by nurses who were beginning to reflect on their work. For many years, nursing practice has been guided by a combination of theoretical frameworks derived from the behavioral and social sciences, the natural sciences, and nursing. This Standard underscores that holistic nurses use theory developed by and applied to nursing. Further, the Standard directs the nurse to use "holistic" nursing theories.

There are many nursing theories in use today.[10,11] Some of these have been with nursing since the 1960s, and some are more recent. Some have been developed as "grand theories," highly abstract and broad in scope. Others—those that have a narrower focus—are referred to as "middle-range theories." A third category, "micro theories," deals with quite narrowly defined phenomena. Some of the "theories" of interest to holistic nurses are better described as philosophies—sets of ideas that describe the meaning of phenomena through analysis, reasoning, and logic.

In keeping with this Standard, the holistic nurse will become familiar with the currently used nursing theories, keeping in mind that every nursing theory purports to be "holistic"—that is, to take into account the client and the nurse as "whole beings" and to guide practice in a manner consistent with holism.

Over the years, AHNA has been asked from time to time to either accept or reject specific theories as "holistic" or not. AHNA has not done this; rather, the view of AHNA has remained one of asking nurses to identify which theory or theories help them best to achieve the goals and/or the kind of practice they believe is most consistent with their view and the client's view of care. This idea is reflected in the following excerpt from AHNA's description of holistic nursing:

> Holistic nursing recognizes that there are two views regarding holism: that holism involves studying and understanding the interrelationships of the bio-psycho-social-spiritual dimensions of the person, recognizing that the whole is greater than the sum of the parts; and that holism involves understanding the individual as an integrated whole interacting with and being acted upon by both internal and external environments. Holistic nursing accepts both views, believing that the goals of holistic nursing can be achieved within either framework. (AHNA, Description of Holistic Nursing, 2000)[12]

While many theories may be used by holistic nurses, there are a few theories or theoretical perspectives that have gained popularity over time. There are theories based on the concept of *caring*: the Philosophy and Science of Caring (Jean Watson) and Cultural Care (Madeline Leininger); theories based on the concept of *relationships* and *adaptation*: the Modeling and Role-Modeling Theory (Helen Erickson, Evelyn Tomlin, and Mary Ann Swain); and theories based on the concept of *energy fields*: the Science of Unitary Human Beings (Martha Rogers), the Theory of Expanding Consciousness (Margaret Newman), and the Theory of Human Becoming (Rosemarie Rizzo Parse). There are two Standards of Practice that address use of nursing theories, each discussed below.

Standard of Practice 2.2.1

Holistic nurses strive to use nursing theories to develop holistic nursing practice and transformational leadership.

Holistic nurses are nurses who think about their practice in efforts to better understand how to meet their client's needs, how to support their client's development, and how to grow as nurses to become experts. Use of theory provides a framework that calls upon each nurse to reflect on his or her practice. For example, for nurses using Watson's theory of Human Care, use of the theory will stimulate thinking about encounters with every client and cause a nurse to ask "In what way did I exhibit unconditional caring toward my clients today? Did my clients experience me as a caring person?" It is this type of reflection on practice that brings each nurse closer to holistic ideals.

Transformational leadership is nursing leadership derived from holistic philosophies.[13] Transformational leadership is a way of providing leadership that is based in collaboration, mutual respect, decision making through discussion and consensus, and emphasis on a fair and just process in organizational behavior. This leadership is "transformational" because those who have experienced it are left changed when the process is over. Thus, transformational leadership changes the individuals as well as the groups and organizations. The holistic principles upon which "transformational" leadership is based are universal human dignity and respect, collaboration, consensus, caring, and process. Table 2–7 summarizes this Standard.

Table 2–7 Nursing and Related Theory

Standard of Practice 2.2.1	*Key Concepts*	*Requisite Knowledge*	*Requisite Skills*
Holistic nurses strive to use nursing theories to develop holistic nursing practice and transformational leadership.	Nursing theories.	Nursing theory, theory development, critiques of theory.	Skills in analysis and reflection.
	Transformational leadership.	Leadership styles, leadership based on holistic principles.	Skills in collaboration, consensus building, and group process.

Nursing Activities

Nursing activities that demonstrate meeting this Standard include: taking classes in nursing theory, reading professional books and journals that describe developments in theory-based practice, attending continuing education sessions in theory, and discussing cases with other nurses from a theoretical perspective. Further, activities where nurses bring a specific theoretical perspective to their work—e.g., incorporate one theory into the practice of an entire unit—also demonstrate meeting this Standard. Lastly, any nurse in a leadership/management role can demonstrate "transformational" leadership by adopting a leadership style based on holistic principles. Such nurses may also be able to influence the practices of an organization to embrace holistic principles in all leadership/management activities.

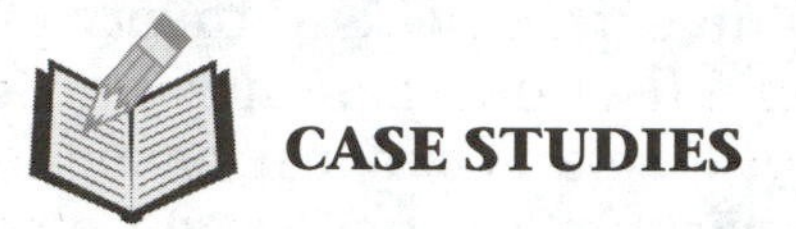

CASE STUDIES

1 Lashan was a nurse working at a busy surgicenter in an urban center in the Southwest. She provided care to clients before and after same-day surgery and was part of a nursing team that met with clients preoperatively to provide orientation to the center and pre-surgery instructions. She became very interested in Watson's theory as a basis for care. She asked her colleagues if they knew of the theory and most of them did, having studied nursing theory in school. Lashan started reflecting on the idea of the "caring encounter" and began to think about her work differently. She recorded a series of cases where she believed that the theory had positively influenced her work. One case was a woman coming in for a hysterectomy, who appeared tearful and frightened. Lashan responded to this client, Mrs. Lewir, by opening herself up to a caring encounter with another human being. Lashan was surprised that Mrs. Lewir immediately responded to her. Mrs. Lewir said she was pleased there was someone there at the surgicenter she could trust, and thanked Lashan for "being there" for her. It appeared that Mrs. Lewir was touched by the fact that Lashan expressed caring. Lashan was unsure if there was really something different or significant about what she herself had done. As she reflected on this case and others, she read about the concept of "healing presence" in a journal, and concluded that caring could be expressed and does have the ability to change the nurse-client relationship in positive ways.

Lashan is meeting this Standard in her practice. She is using a theory, reflecting on her practice, and growing in her ability to help clients in the process.

2 George, a family nurse practitioner, practiced in a rural area with a group of three other nurse practitioners and two family physicians. He saw a range of patients each day, attended to their immediate medical needs, and also took time to uncover any family or social situations that might prohibit his clients from obtaining services or adhering to the prescribed treatments. His care was compassionate, and he tried to do the best for each person or family he saw.

He did not use a nursing theory in his practice—he stated that he learned theories in school, but in the real world one had to practice in a manner consistent with others in the practice and dependent upon what was reimbursed through third parties.

Theory is not relevant to George. He is not meeting this Standard as he is not using a theory to provide a basis for reflection.

Standard of Practice 2.2.2

Holistic nurses interpret, use, and document information relevant to a person's care according to a theoretical framework.

Documentation of care according to a theory can be done in one of two ways: the nurse may use the language of the theory to describe the client situations or the nurse may use one of the standard classifications of nursing phenomena (for example, the NANDA or Omaha lists) and write the theory perspective in the "related to" clause that follows the diagnosis. Either way it is possible for one reading the record to understand the theory perspective and know that the nurse's work is grounded in theory. Such recording provides evidence of theory-based practice and also encourages the use of theory by others reading the record. Table 2–8 summarizes this Standard. The Case Studies provide sample records of charting below.

Table 2–8 Documentation According to Theory

Standard of Practice 2.2.2	*Key Concepts*	*Requisite Knowledge*	*Requisite Skills*
Holistic nurses interpret, use, and document information relevant to a person's care according to a theoretical framework.	Interpret, use, and document information.	Nursing and related theories.	Synthesis of theory and practice.
	Theoretical framework.	Documentation systems. Recordkeeping.	Literacy required for documentation.

Nursing Activities

Nursing activities that demonstrate Standard 2.2.2 include both the use of theory and the ability to select and use a documentation system that reflects the theoretical perspective in client care.

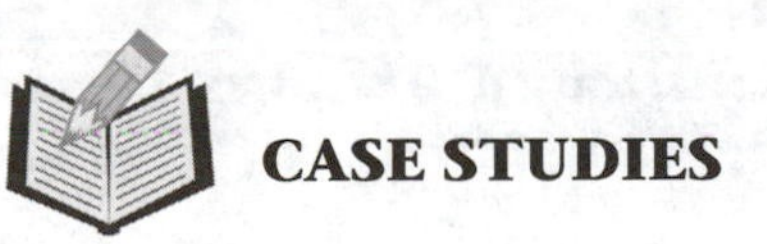

CASE STUDIES

1 Nurse Valerie was giving care to a client in an outpatient setting at a senior resource center. An elderly woman, Mrs. Rose, came to see Valerie and described "not feeling well today" and "not being my usual self." Upon further discussion, Valerie learned that Mrs. Rose was worried about her husband, who was being treated for hypertension and was not responding well to treatment. Mrs. Rose expressed concern that he might be seriously ill and she might not be able to care for him. She expressed being in a state of worry, not being able to sleep at night, and not knowing where to go for help. Mrs. Rose said that Valerie was the only person she had been able to talk to about the problem. Valerie was interpreting Mrs. Rose's concerns from within the Modeling and Role-Modeling theory. As directed by the theory, she asked Mrs. Rose what she needed from the nurse and the center. Mrs. Rose said that she needed a place to come during the day and a phone number of someone with whom she could talk at night, if needed. Valerie recorded two individual nursing diagnoses, according to the NANDA list:

Anxiety r/t a state of arousal secondary to the illness of spouse.
Sleep pattern disturbance: unable to sleep at night, r/t stress state.

Valerie's statements of nursing diagnoses identified the nursing concerns she and Mrs. Rose worked together to address. Her "related to" clauses identify specific states in the Adaptive Potential Assessment Model (APAM) that are expressed within the Modeling and Role-Modeling theory.[14] Thus, in keeping with this Standard, her diagnostic statements identified the theory.

2 Kim worked with a client on an oncology unit. Samantha S. had just had a mastectomy for breast cancer. Samantha was first day post-op, having some pain and discomfort but able, she said, to handle herself. She expressed concerns that "it is hard to believe that the surgery has really happened. . . Everything went so quickly." Samantha had been reassured by her physician that the surgery went well and complete recovery was expected. Samantha was quiet on the unit, and when her relatives (husband and sister) came to visit, she looked away from them and told them she was tired. Kim, who was also using the Modeling and Role-Modeling Theory, assessed that Samantha was in a state of impoverishment. She recorded the following:

Mrs. S. has expressed concerns related to her perception that the diagnosis, treatment, and surgery went too quickly. Mrs. S. states: "It's hard to believe the surgery really happened." Mrs. S. remains resting in bed, with little obvious energy to interact with family visitors. Assessment: state of impoverishment. Care: provide direct physical care and emotional support at this time.

Kim's records indicated what she observed and demonstrated that the care is grounded in a theory—the language in her assessment, as well as Valerie's, is derived from the APAM model. Kim's records are consistent with Standard 2.2.2.

2.3 HOLISTIC NURSING AND RELATED RESEARCH

■■ Holistic nurses provide care and guidance to persons through nursing interventions and holistic therapies consistent with research findings and other sound evidence. ■■

Research is an essential component of all professional nursing practice. The nurse must have a good understanding of research concepts and methods, be able to read research publications, and understand the meaning of research findings. Care must be grounded in what is known, and clients must be given valid information from which to make decisions regarding their treatment plans.

Thus, holistic nurses must read publications that keep them informed about the status of treatments, modalities, and interventions thought to be helpful in specific areas of practice. The nurse must be current in the nursing and medical science related to his or her particular area of practice, and must also be current regarding any holistic therapies that he/she brings into practice. Skills expected of the nurse include: knowledge of research designs, both qualitative and quantitative; skills in critical thinking and critical reading; understanding of statistics; and ability to interpret findings for application to practice. There are six Standards that relate to research.

Standard of Practice 2.3.1

Holistic nurses use available research and evidence from different explanatory models to mutually create a plan of care with a person.

Standard of Practice 2.3.2

Holistic nurses use expert clinical judgment to select appropriate nursing interventions.

Holistic nurses must use research findings and evidence derived from research when planning care. Further, the holistic nurse must understand differing explanatory models—different ways of thinking and different ways of knowing—to be able to provide a complete resource to clients about care and treatments.

The scientific controlled clinical trial has been the "gold standard" of evidence in medical treatment. These clinical trials involve very large group studies evaluating treatments using experimental and control groups in settings that either are or closely resemble real life. Once a treatment has been found to be useful in the controlled clinical trial, offering that treatment to all is thought to be appropriate. Evidence-based practice, the current trend in health care, depends on having knowledge derived from the controlled clinical trial.

The emphasis in medical care on the experimental study and the traditions of biomedical science that were passed along to nursing led nurses to initially conduct all studies from a quantitative and experimental approach. As nursing developed as a field and discipline of its own, nurses became more and more interested in aspects of care, caring, and treatments that could not be studied through the traditional quantitative methods of biomedical science. Thus, nurses learned about and adopted research methods from other disciplines: phenomenology from philosophy, grounded theory from sociology, and ethnography from anthropology.[15] Nurses developed expertise in qualitative research, the purpose of which is to focus on the lived experience or the subjective experience of persons undergoing a specific condition or treatment. More than likely, it is the intimacy with which nurses interact with clients that led nurses to pursue a qualitative approach to research.

Today, nursing researchers use many differing research approaches to study the phenomena of nursing. Nurses conduct surveys to learn about populations; nurses manage clinical trials to evaluate treatment interventions; nurses study the cultural values of health within defined groups; nurses document and describe the lived experience of clients with many differing health care problems. Each of these research approaches has value, and all are needed to advance nursing's work.

Holistic nurses must appreciate the many kinds of research methods and approaches currently available. The nurse must read published reports of research and be able to describe to the client what is known and not known about treatments and interventions in order to work with the client to plan care. Table 2–9 summarizes Standards 2.3.1 and 2.3.2.

Table 2–9 Use of Research

Standards of Practice 2.3.1 and 2.3.2	*Key Concepts*	*Requisite Knowledge*	*Requisite Skills*
Holistic nurses use available research and evidence from different explanatory models to mutually create a plan of care with a person, and use expert clinical judgment to select appropriate nursing interventions.	Evidence. Explanatory models. Mutually plan care. Expert clinical judgment to plan care.	Research methods and interpretations.	Critical thinking. Analysis of evidence.

Nursing Activities

Activities that support these Standards include: reading published reports and journals to keep up to date and current in topics related to one's work; distinguishing between research findings and reports based on opinion or experience; analyzing results and recommendations for applicability to one's own practice; and establishing time to talk with clients about mutually determined goals and plans of care.

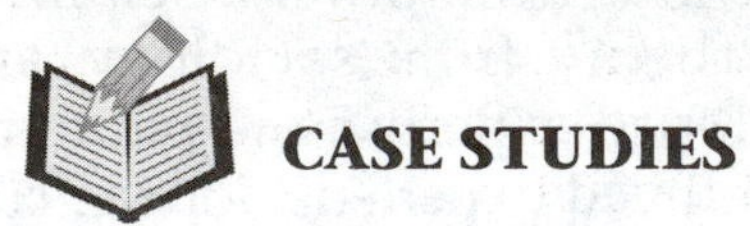

CASE STUDIES

1 Marshella was a nurse working on an acute care unit in a large urban hospital. Many of the clients she saw were young men in acute sickle cell crisis.

Her experience with these clients validated her view that clients experiencing sickle cell crisis experience pain, and because the condition is one that does recur, she noted that her clients tended to come into the unit not only in pain, but also experiencing anxiety about the pain. To Marshella and many of her clients, pain relief/provision of comfort was a very high nursing priority.

Marshella read a great deal about the condition of sickle cell crisis, and she also read many published reports on pain control. She noted from her readings that pain among clients with this condition is common and often not well controlled. She also learned that in studies of physicians and nurses, health care professionals seem to underplay the degree of pain experienced by these clients.[16,17] Further, in published reports about pain control in general, research has indicated that nurses have not considered pain management of high priority.[18] Some have even concluded that patients' experience of pain is a commonly neglected area of nursing care.

Analyzing the available research, Marshella concluded that she needed to talk with her clients regarding their own experience of pain, and ask them if they thought alternate forms of pain control (distraction, music, TT, imagery) might be helpful in addition to medication. Further, in thinking about what was known and not known about this condition, Marshella noted that there was no research on the experience of this particular condition based on the cultural perspective of African-American males, or Caribbean males. She concluded that the next step in caring for these clients would be to initiate or support research from an ethnographic perspective on the experience and meaning of living with sickle cell anemia and entering the hospital in sickle cell crisis.

Marshella is meeting this Standard—she is using available research findings in her practice, and she is identifying the areas of research that are needed to obtain better data on how to assist this client population.[19]

2 Jeanne, a nurse working in the same hospital as Marshella, cared for patients on the oncology unit. Many of her clients were patients with metastatic tumors undergoing chemotherapy and radiation treatments. For some, palliative care alone was being offered.

Jeanne was a conscientious nurse, careful in her work. She followed the hospital policies and procedures and attended continuing education offerings in oncology. She was not a member of the Oncology Nursing Association and did not subscribe to *Oncology Nursing Forum,* so she did not read the journal in her area of practice on a regular basis at all. In fact, she only read this (or any other) journal when someone at work brought an article in and said "Look at this! This is what we ought to be doing here."

Jeanne designed plans of care for her clients based on their stated needs and her best judgments about what to do for them. She used good judgment in planning care that was appropriate and caring. She found that, over time, she used many of the same interventions and approaches and that her interventions worked for the most part with a majority of patients. She believed that there are always some clients whose needs cannot be met.

Jeanne is not meeting this Standard—she is either unable or unwilling to use research findings in her practice. Jeanne is practicing nursing at a basic, legally defensible level, but she is not practicing professional nursing.

Standard of Practice 2.3.3

Holistic nurses discuss holistic application to clinical situations where rigorous research has not been done.

There are many areas of nursing practice in which research has not been done, or for which there is only a small number of completed research projects. Holistic nurses must discuss what is known and not known about care situations and make their best judgments on how to proceed with limited information. Many nurses analyze these situations on the basis of how critical the need is for new or different treatments or interventions and how invasive or benign is the treatment or intervention being offered. Clearly, the nurse has a mandate to "do no harm." Incorporating research findings into practice too early or generalizing beyond the scope of the findings has the potential to "do harm." However, if the treatment or intervention being considered is noninvasive and harmless, there is better justification to implement the treatment, while collecting data to evaluate its effectiveness. Table 2–10 summarizes this Standard.

Table 2–10 Application: Research to Practice

Standard of Practice 2.3.3	*Key Concepts*	*Requisite Knowledge*	*Requisite Skills*
Holistic nurses discuss application to clinical situations where rigorous research has not been done.	Application to practice. Rigorous research.	Understanding of research methods and data. Knowledge of generalizability of research findings.	Critical thinking skills. Analytical skills.

Nursing Activities

Nursing activities that meet this Standard include analysis of research data, making critical decisions regarding application to practice, and discussing the potential benefits and risks of introducing new treatments/interventions into practice with other nurses.

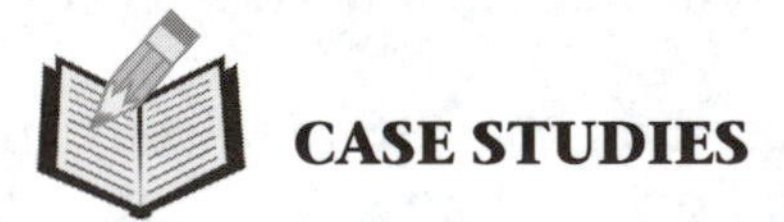

CASE STUDIES

1 Bob was a nurse working with a population of college students who described being unable to sleep at night due to worries about classes, homework, tests, etc. Bob knew of published research on the use of music therapy (tape-recorded music) that helped elderly patients with sleep-pattern disturbances in a home setting. This research utilized a small sample and could be described as a pilot study. The results could not be generalized to a younger population with very different life circumstances than the elderly in the study. However, the intervention (listening to tape-recorded music at the hour of sleep and again during the night if awakened) was harmless, the intervention could easily be made part of the clients' routines (college students have access to tapes and headsets), and the tapes of soothing music could easily be made on Bob's campus. He discussed the idea of offering prerecorded tapes at a team meeting of nurses in the health center. They reasoned that even if there were no data on the use of this intervention with college students, there was potential for benefit and there were virtually no risks involved. Bob offered the tapes to students who expressed having sleep disturbances, explaining to the clients the level of knowledge (or lack thereof) and the potential benefits of this experiment. Bob found that a great majority of his student clients wanted to "try out" the music approach before doing anything else as a workup for sleep disturbance.

Bob's actions are in keeping with this Standard. He is cautious about applying findings outside of what the evidence suggests, he discusses his ideas about the modality with others, and he makes a professionally defensible suggestion to his clients. Further, he ensures that his clients have enough information to make an informed choice about using music for their own sleep disturbances.

2 Gina was a nurse who also worked in college health. She was seeing a group of students who had cold symptoms. Gina decided to set up a "Care for Your Cold Center" to provide information to students about how to manage their cold symptoms themselves. She provided information on the need for adequate rest, fluids (with hot tea and chicken soup recommended), Vitamin C, hot showers, and echinacea as the "best" treatments for the common cold. Gina had not investigated the research base for these treatments—they were interventions she had used herself for colds and found to be helpful. She discussed these interventions with others who had used them, and her group of friends all agreed that her list of interventions belonged at the "Care for Your Cold Center."

Gina's actions are not in keeping with this Standard. Not only has she not evaluated the research base of what she is providing, but she did not discuss the applications of these interventions in a professional manner with anyone before setting up her center. (Had she completed even a basic review of available research, she would have encountered data on the use of zinc for cold treatment. These data, as incomplete and imperfect as they are, would have been something she could have considered on the basis of known facts.)

Standard of Practice 2.3.4

Holistic nurses create an environment conducive to systematic inquiry into healing and health issues by engaging in research or supporting and utilizing the research of others.

To advance the science of holistic nursing, it is essential that all nurses help to create work and practice environments supportive to research. This means that all nurses should be willing to participate in research projects whenever the opportunity arises, and should be supportive to the ideas that others have about conducting studies and evaluating research findings. While it is true that only a small number of holistic nurses will have careers as nurse researchers, all will be able to support the research process in some way. Table 2–11 presents a summary of this Standard.

Table 2–11 Environment Conducive to Inquiry

Standard of Practice 2.3.4	*Key Concepts*	*Requisite Knowledge*	*Requisite Skills*
Holistic nurses create an environment conducive to systematic inquiry into healing and health issues by engaging in research or supporting and utilizing the research of others.	Environments conducive to research. Use of research in practice. Engaging in research.	Research process. Organizational behaviors.	Acceptance of the research process. Valuing the role of research in advancing holistic nursing.

Nursing Activities

For nurses not directly involved in conducting research, activities such as attending network meetings to evaluate cases using research, participation in hospital "nursing rounds," volunteering to serve on research committees, and willingness to serve as research subjects/informants demonstrate commitment to this Standard. Also, nurses who support research can do so informally through the use of conversation about the value of research. By verbally stating that research is needed and valuable (often as a counter to negative statements made about research), nurses can be instrumental in the way that research is viewed by a particular work group. Lastly, nurses can create a work environment where research findings are applied to practice through discussion of research applicable to the specific practice setting and willingness to update policies and procedures based on evidence.

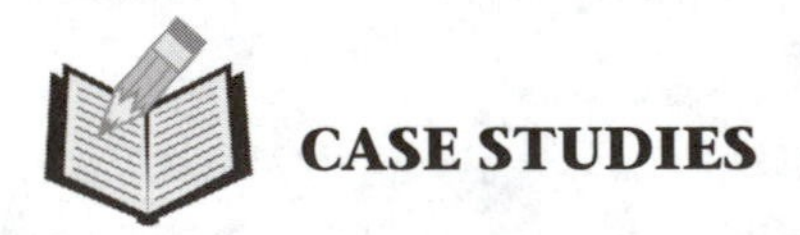

CASE STUDIES

1 June was working as a charge nurse in an endocrine clinic with patients who were primarily diabetic. A nurse researcher approached her and discussed plans for a project to evaluate the degree to which adherence to prescribed regimes was affected by specific factors at home. The nurse researcher had been interested in this topic for some time and had already conducted a small pilot study. The researcher planned an investigation that included both qualitative and quantitative work. June would have to make some alterations in the scheduling of patients to help make the clients available on clinic days to the researcher. She would also have to give the research nurse access to a conference room that would otherwise be used by nursing staff taking breaks.

June was very busy and, in all honesty, the thought of making time for a research project on her unit was unwelcome. However, June was committed to the use of research and had to admit she was even intrigued about the qualitative part of the study. Deciding to do all she could to aid the nurse researcher's success, she gave the project her full support. Further, she explained to her staff that the use of the room once a week was a small contribution they could make to nursing research and presented the idea to them in the most positive light.

June is meeting this Standard because she is being supportive of the research effort. While she is busy and at least to some degree the research study is an intrusion on her time and the time of her staff, she is willing to assist the researcher. Further, June creates an environment conducive to research when she interprets the events to her staff in a positive, rather than negative, manner.

Standard of Practice 2.3.5

Holistic nurses disseminate research findings at meetings and through publications to further develop the foundation and practice of holistic nursing.

Standard of Practice 2.3.6

Holistic nurses provide consultation services on holistic nursing interventions to persons and communities based on research.

Together, these Standards speak to the development of the roles of nurse researcher and nurse consultant. These roles are taken on by those holistic nurses with advanced skills in research and extensive knowledge of published research. More than likely, nurses assuming these roles will be doctorally prepared nurses with considerable expertise in research. Other nurses can participate in these endeavors, particularly the consultative process, if working along with an expert nurse researcher. Table 2–12 presents a summary of these Standards.

Table 2–12 Dissemination of Research Findings/Consultation Regarding Findings

Standards of Practice 2.3.5 and 2.3.6	*Key Concepts*	*Requisite Knowledge*	*Requisite Skills*
Holistic nurses disseminate research findings at meetings and through	Disseminate research findings.	Expert knowledge of research methods and interpretation of findings.	Critical thinking skills.

continues

Table 2–12 continued

Standards of Practice 2.3.5 and 2.3.6	*Key Concepts*	*Requisite Knowledge*	*Requisite Skills*
publications to further develop the foundation and practice of holistic nursing and provide consultation services on holistic nursing interventions to persons and communities based on research.	Consult on the use of research findings.	Familiarity with a wide range of published studies.	Analytical skills. Ability to work with groups in consultation. Writing skills needed for publication. Communication skills for presentations to both lay and professional groups.

Nursing Activities

The activities that demonstrate meeting these Standards are the activities of a nurse researcher. Publishing findings of one's own work, critiquing studies done by others, reading publications regularly to remain current in the field, and speaking to nursing and other groups on the results of research are essential activities of a researcher. One with this advanced knowledge is also in a position to share expertise with communities and groups who have a need to understand research findings for their own care. Lastly, a nurse at this level should also make himself or herself available to the public media whenever the media shows an interest in a particular type of research.

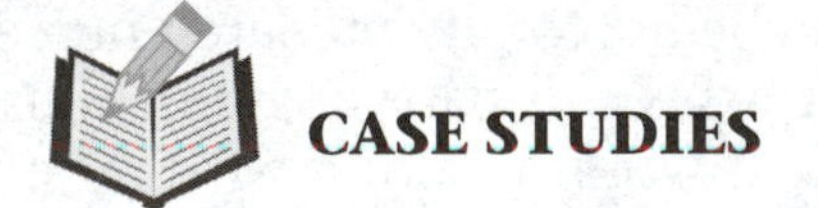

CASE STUDIES

1 Mary Ellen, a nurse researcher, has completed a study on the use of pet therapy in a socialization group for persons with Alzheimer's disease at a senior resource center. She has found that clients increase their interactions with each other and with the staff if a group of puppies is brought into the sessions. Her work is an extension of previous work in the topic. She has published her findings in a nursing journal and has been asked to speak on the topic to members of the local Kennel Club. While speaking at the Kennel Club is not a typical method of disseminating nursing research, Mary Ellen believes that this invitation gives her a chance to speak about holism in health care and the use of pet-assisted therapy to a wide range of citizens in her community. She accepts the invitation to speak and introduces nearly 100 interested citizens to a very new view of nursing. Her actions are in keeping with Standards 2.3.5 and 2.3.6.

2 Richard is a faculty member at a School of Nursing. He has an extensive background in ethnographic research and has studied members of the urban community in which he lives for the past six years. He has published several papers resulting from his research and is becoming nationally known in nursing for his work. He has been asked to consult with a group of nurses from another state on how to set up visiting nurse services to an urban, inner-city population. He willingly accepts this invitation and travels to their offices to discuss his work and the relevance of his and other research findings to their practice. His actions are in keeping with these Standards because he is willing to consult with others about his work and travels to assist them in applying his research findings to practice.

CONCLUSION

Core Value 2 covers a range of topics. Taken together, these topics call upon the nurse to reflect on care and to engage in thoughtful, considered practice. Ethics provides the grounding in the essence of holism—caring, compassion, respect, and dignity. Theory provides the framework for thoughtful practice and communication about practice. Research provides the basis for credibility of practice, the ability to study and learn about the effectiveness and benefits of nursing care. Ethics, Theory, and Research each impact on practice while helping to move the profession forward. These three concepts are foundational to holism and are presented in the Standards as essential elements of professional practice.

NOTES

1. J. Watson, *Nursing: Human Science and Human Care—A Theory of Nursing* (New York: NLN Press, 1988).
2. American Holistic Nurses' Association, *Code of Ethics for Holistic Nursing Practice* (Flagstaff, AZ: AHNA, 1992).
3. P. Benner, *The Primacy of Caring* (Menlo Park, CA: Addison-Wesley, 1989).
4. J.R. Ellis and C.L. Hartley, *Nursing in Today's World* (Philadelphia: J.B. Lippincott Co., 1999).
5. American Holistic Nurses' Association, *Position Statement in Support of a Healthful Environment* (Flagstaff, AZ: AHNA, 1992).
6. American Holistic Nurses' Association, *Position Statement on Social Issues* (Flagstaff, AZ: AHNA, 1992).
7. M. Burkhardt and A. Nathaniel, *Ethics and Issues in Contemporary Nursing* (Albany, NY: Delmar Publishers, 1998), 40–47.
8. Burkhardt and Nathaniel, *Ethics and Issues in Contemporary Nursing*, 53–56.
9. L. Frisch, "Ethical and Legal Bases for Care," in *Psychiatric Mental Health Nursing*, eds. N. Frisch and L. Frisch (Albany, NY: Delmar Publishers, 1998), 131–144.
10. A. Marriner-Tomey and M.R. Alligood, *Nurse Theorists and Their Work*, 4th ed. (St. Louis: Mosby, 1997).
11. J. George, ed., *Nursing Theories: The Base for Professional Nursing*, 4th ed. (Norwalk, CT: Appleton & Lange, 1995).
12. American Holistic Nurses' Association, *Description of Holistic Nursing* (Flagstaff, AZ: AHNA, 2000).

13. J. Koerner, "Reflections: Transformational Leadership," in *Journal of Holistic Nursing* 16 (1998): 223–226.
14. N. Frisch and S. Bowman, "Helen Erickson, Evelyn Tomlin and Mary Ann Swain," in *Nursing Theories: The Base for Professional Nursing*, 4th ed., ed. J. George (Norwalk, CT: Appleton & Lange, 1995), 355–372.
15. N. Burns and S. Grove, *Understanding Nursing Research*, 2d ed. (Philadelphia: W.B. Saunders, 1999), 337–377.
16. J. Alleyne and V. Thomas, "The Management of Sickle Cell Crisis Pain as Experienced by Patients and Their Carers," *Journal of Advanced Nursing* 19 (1994): 725–732.
17. B. Shapiro et al., "Sickle Cell–Related Pain: Perceptions of Medical Practitioners," *Journal of Pain and Symptom Management* 14 (1997): 168–174.
18. D. Brockopp et al., "Barriers to Change: A Pain Management Project," *International Journal of Nursing Studies* 35 (1998): 226–232.
19. The author gratefully acknowledges the work of Colleen McInnis, SN, of Cleveland State University who developed this case study.

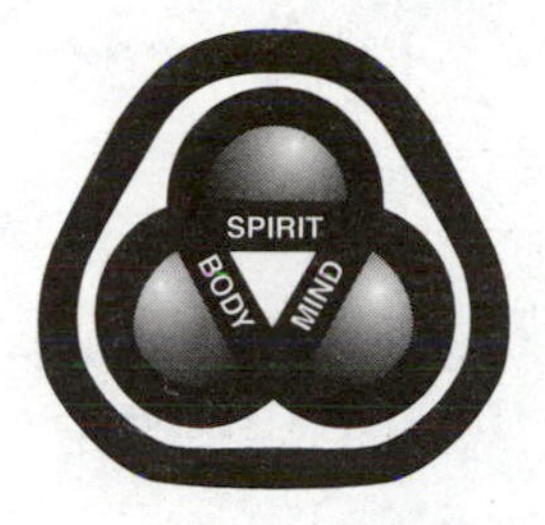

CORE VALUE 3

HOLISTIC NURSE SELF-CARE

Johanne A. Quinn

3.1 Holistic Nurse Self-Care

Holistic nurses engage in self-care and further develop their own personal awareness as being an instrument of healing to better serve self and others.

Self-care is a vital concept to the practice of holistic nursing. As a Core Value, it underscores the importance of self-understanding and self-reflection so that one may ultimately become more aware and understanding of the human experience of others. Conceptually, self-care is rooted within the realm of personal responsibility for health and it is an essential expression of individual freedom and self-determination. When viewed within a wellness framework, self-care implies personal choice and self-initiated actions, meaning the health behaviors one chooses for self are based on personal values and one's understanding of the meaning of health.[1] Foster and Janssens noted that in Orem's conceptual model of nursing, self-care is defined by showing that one's behavior is directed toward self or environment to freely regulate factors that affect development and functioning in decisions of one's life, health, or well-being.[2] In the holistic caring model, self-care is defined within the framework of wellness and whole person care. In this theory, individuals are taught to meet their self-care needs by seeking balance and harmony between their physiological, psychological, emotional, and spiritual self. This balance and harmony is guided by an awareness of self, society, nature, and the universe.[3]

The holistic nurse, as instrument of healing, uses unconditional presence in creating an environment to guide and support the healing process. With attention and intention, the environment becomes one in which the client can feel safe to explore the dimensions of self in the healing moment. By partnering with the client in the healing journey, the nurse provides opportunity to exchange energy, truth, and communication with clients while fostering their attunement to their own healing capacities.[4,5] Accordingly, when applying the concepts of self-care to practice, holistic nurses support the client's choice for self-care strategies and healing paths, and they clearly avoid substituting professional authority. The nurse's primary goal is to assist clients in reaching their highest level of participation in all self-care activities.

Standard of Practice 3.1.1

Holistic nurses recognize that a person's body-mind-spirit has healing capacities that can be enhanced and supported through self-care practices.

This Standard highlights the many facets of Psychophysiology, Psychoneuroimmunology, and Self-Regulation Theory, which support holistic interventions drawing on both proven and intuitive knowledge.[3] By engaging clients in activities aimed at understanding body-mind-spirit interconnectedness, healing can improve markedly.[6] Clients become aware of their inner strengths and adopt effective coping styles and strategies, thus altering activities at the cellular level, and disease processes are reversed.[7,8,9] This Standard clearly dictates the importance of integrating knowledge from the sciences, using holistic interventions, developing critical thinking skills related to a holistic paradigm of care, and planning future research to document client outcomes related to body-mind healing.

Table 3–1 illustrates the nursing knowledge and skill required for a nurse to meet Standard 3.1.1.

Table 3–1 Honoring the Healing Capacities of Self-Care

Standard of Practice 3.1.1	*Key Concepts*	*Requisite Knowledge*	*Requisite Skills*
Holistic nurses recognize that a person's body-mind-spirit has healing capacities that can be enhanced and supported through self-care practices.	Healing capacity of humankind.	Knowledge of body-mind connections and principles of wholeness; energy field healing; health promotion models.	Ability to integrate knowledge and skills from the humanities, sciences, and nursing.
	Body-mind-spirit connectedness.	Knowledge of self-regulation theory; principles of psychophysiology and psychoneuro-immunology; concepts related to the circle of human potential.	Ability to demonstrate human caring and relationship skills; supporting health locus of control.
	Self-care practices.	Knowledge of holistic models of health-care delivery; patterns and processes of physical and psychological human functioning.	Ability to perform a holistic health assessment and clinical intervention skills; ability to facilitate healing in self and others.

Nursing Activities

Nursing actions that demonstrate this Standard include the use of alternative therapies as a complement to conventional nursing care techniques. One example is the use of stress assessment techniques along with exploring and learning relaxation strategies, imagery, meditation, psychotherapy, prayer, therapeutic touch, art, dance, and music.[3] Therapeutic presence involves centering, meditating, demonstrating intentionality, keeping open and intuitive, communicating, loving, and connecting.[5] Caring and interpersonal relationships are developed by demonstrating genuine regard, such as knowing the client and developing an ability to collaborate or partner with the client to meet his/her self-care needs independent of any coercion.[10] Communicating is the human response pattern of talking, listening, and using reflective feedback.[10] Problem solving and diagnostic reasoning involve making clinical judgments based on the integration of pertinent data from multiple sources.[11] Clarifying values uses strategies of discovery for choosing, prizing, and acting on matters of important significance.[3] Advocacy is interceding or acting on behalf of the client to provide the highest quality of care possible.[12] Healing awareness is a conscious recognition and a focusing of attention on sensations, feelings, conditions, and facts dealing with needs of self and others.[13]

CASE STUDIES

1 Sonja was an active 60-year-old admitted to the hospital for elective surgery for a total knee replacement following several falls and injuries. After Nurse Marsha completed the admission history, she was preparing to review postoperative medications and leg exercises using whirlpool therapy. When Sonja and Marsha began talking, it became very evident that Sonja had prepared for this surgery by using guided imagery. She explained how she spent many weeks imagining the surgeon's knife as an instrument of healing rather than considering the blade as causing an assault on her knee. Sonja declined the medication because of the benefits of her imagery. Marsha conveyed an acceptance and full understanding of Sonja's self-care activities, realizing that Sonja had engaged the full power of her imagination to cope with the postoperative pain.

Marsha met Standard 3.1.1 because she supported Sonja and did not attempt to coerce her into accepting medications postoperatively.

2 Emilio was a 35-year-old admitted to the hospital for hernia repair. On his first postoperative day, he was intently listening to music and was in a very peaceful state. Beth, his nurse, came into his room to take vital signs; she abruptly turned the music off, then grabbed Emilio's arm to apply the blood pressure cuff. She went on to explain that she was very busy and the only nurse on the unit. Emilio was startled by this sudden action on Beth's part and seemed disturbed that his concentration had been broken.

Beth does not meet Standard 3.1.1 because she failed to realize that Emilio was using music as a therapy to create an atmosphere of quiet calm. His breathing was normal and he was showing no signs of pain, restlessness, discomfort, or anxiety. Had Beth learned the Art of Caring, she would not have interrupted Emilio in this quiet moment; she could have returned at a later time to check vital signs.

Standard of Practice 3.1.2

Holistic nurses identify and integrate self-care strategies to enhance their physical, psychological, sociological, and spiritual well-being.

Staying healthy or taking care of one's health problems is a fundamental need that underscores one's responsibility for his/her own life, health, and well-being. This Standard dictates that holistic nurses embrace health-promoting activities and engage in health-protecting behaviors for self as well as in setting goals and planning care for others. This includes making lifestyle changes and maximizing one's potential to prevent disease. Yet, for most people, changing behaviors that are counterproductive to good health is often difficult. Studies have shown that changing to a healthier lifestyle may only occur as the result of illness or in response to a specific treatment regime.[14] However, when the motivation to initiate the healthier activities is internalized and genuinely made on one's own behalf, the goal is more likely to be accomplished. A recent study showed that lifestyle change was more successful and longer lasting when individuals were actively involved in devising, implementing, evaluating, and revising their own plans for change.[15]

This Standard also emphasizes the need to ensure the good health and well-being of the whole person. It means he/she has to balance that part of self that relates to not only the physical but also the emotional and spiritual needs. Choosing self-care strategies must incorporate knowledge of mind-body environmental interactions and their influences on health. Personal values and a sense of life's purpose are critical to success in goal setting, improving personal experiences, and making deliberate choices for wellness-promoting behaviors used daily. It might sound like a cliché, but caring for self does give one energy to care for others.

Table 3–2 illustrates the nursing knowledge and skill required for a nurse to meet Standard 3.1.2.

Table 3–2 Nurturing the Healing Capacities of Self-Care

Standard of Practice 3.1.2	*Key concepts*	*Requisite Knowledge*	*Requisite Skills*
Holistic nurses identify and integrate self-care strategies to enhance their physical,	Physical self-care strategies.	Nursing knowledge related to health promotion, maintenance, and restoration.	A willingness to engage in health-promoting and health-protecting behaviors.

continues

Table 3–2 continued

Standard of Practice 3.1.2	*Key concepts*	*Requisite Knowledge*	*Requisite Skills*
psychological, sociological, and spiritual well-being.	Psychological self-care strategies.	Knowledge of theories of self-reflection, body-mind communication; knowledge relating to expressing emotions appropriately and effectively.	Empowering self to modify attitudes and behaviors to develop healthy life patterns; ability to assess and recognize personal feelings and emotions.
	Sociological self-care strategies.	Nursing knowledge related to social responsibility and sense of community, supporting concepts of global health and improving economic factors.	Ability to create and participate in satisfying relationships; use wellness programs to promote support systems, create social networks, and make lifestyle changes.
	Spiritual well-being.	Scientific knowledge related to awareness of higher levels of consciousness; understanding that beliefs and feelings are tools and powers of healing.	Ability to develop a religious belief and faith in a higher power; to deliver compassionate care; to increase faith-support resources; to engage in activities to awaken the inner spirit.

Nursing Activities

Nursing actions that demonstrate this Standard include: promoting balance between physical, emotional, and spiritual needs; increasing knowledge about oneself; developing health promotion goals that can be realistically achieved in six months; taking an active role to improve health; enjoying a basic sense of well-being; developing a personal health/fitness plan.

Balancing personal needs requires positive thinking. It also requires one to create positive expectations for health, healing, peace, and tranquility. By increasing self-knowledge, nurses gain an inner wisdom of what it means to be human. This increased self-awareness guides one to become more aware and understanding of the experiences of others.[16] An important outcome of learning to care for self is that nurses learn the value of therapeutic measures such as the use of humor to release stress and how friendship and love enrich one's being.[17] More importantly, the nurse learns to think well of himself/herself, realizing that a good self-image is the foundation of good health. Further, staying healthy requires that one integrate health promotion goals into one's individual health patterns. In general, individuals must figure out, based on what they enjoy and will keep doing, how to fulfill their physical self-care needs and their mental self-care needs and what they will do to care for their spiritual self. Individuals need to motivate themselves to modify attitudes and behaviors and to develop healthy life patterns.

Setting realistic goals and maintaining consistency in what one does is most important. While these principles are very basic, they are often the most neglected concepts when nurses develop a plan of self-care. For example, designing a wellness program that focuses on maintaining good nutritional habits such as eating a well-balanced, low-fat diet of wholesome food will obviously help to keep one energetic and free of illnesses, but a healthy diet is not enough. Nurses, like many others, need to convince themselves that even moderate exercise makes a huge difference both in how they feel and what illnesses they get.

Mental well-being requires that one integrate pleasurable activities into one's daily life. Nurses need to develop coping strategies to control stress and to feel good about who they are. One's daily routine should include the use of relaxation techniques and/or personal activities that help with relaxation. Further, one's life patterns should include plenty of wholesome leisure activities. For example, strategies used throughout the day could include taking naps, relaxing while eating meals, playing with one's children or grandchildren, and/or caring for a pet.

Spiritual well-being is also an outcome when one acknowledges the inner core. Studies have shown that faith, prayer, and spiritual beliefs can play an important role in health, healing, and recovery from illness.[18] When nurses learn to integrate the use of spiritual images through visualization and/or use of affirmations in their daily practice, they maintain a daily awareness of higher levels of consciousness. Of equal importance to a sense of spiritual wellness is the acceptance that calm and serenity start with oneself. Often nurses must overcome personal trials and tribulations they cannot change. At such times, it is important to use measures such as seeking consensus to resolve issues, at work or at home, to promote peace in one's internal and/or external environment.

CASE STUDIES

1 Jasmine is a nurse who lives in a family supportive of self-care. Family members purposefully take time each evening before dinner for quiet rest or what they call "peaceful time." When one of the family members has had a bad day, he/she tells the family. Other family members agree that it is their role to be the support. They take over all the chores and allow the member who has had a bad day additional time to unwind and relax. Others prepare the evening meal and they eat with a sense of peace. This family is practicing self-care in a collaborative way.

2 Hunter is a nurse and a devout Christian man. He prays before going to work to seek assistance from God and to provide support for the spiritual health of his clients. With all difficult situations at work, Hunter prays for spiritual guidance. He observes his clients and their response to illness or tragedy. He willingly prays with his clients to assist them to cope with their pain. Hunter believes his spiritual connecting with God provides him with a sense of serenity at work.

3 Nurse Renee is an intensive care nurse who works 12-hour shifts. She has many additional responsibilities, including keeping up with the school work for her BSN degree, transporting her children to after-school activities, and entertaining at church functions to meet responsibilities of being a minister's wife. Renee is in the fast lane! She goes to bed at night upset and crying that everything was not done impeccably. Renee does not meet Standard 3.1.2 because she has not learned how to develop coping strategies to control stress and to feel good about who she is and the daily achievements she does have.

Standard of Practice 3.1.3

Holistic nurses recognize and address at-risk health patterns and begin the process of change.

This Standard clearly emphasizes the need to initiate programs aimed at eliminating risks associated with obesity, lack of exercise, or other health hazards such as smoking, excessive use of alcohol, or consuming drugs or high amounts of caffeine. This Standard also underscores the need to be equally concerned about the importance of immunizations, driving safely, safe sex, and firearm safety in one's home. As holistic nurses, a corresponding quality is the need to be emotionally free of stress when trying to care for others. This creates the need to learn how to handle stressful events at home, at school, at work, and in the community in nonconfrontational ways. Furthermore, it encourages one to improve one's external environment, social relationships, support systems, and, for some, their economic situation.

As health care providers, holistic nurses learn that health improvement begins with awareness and grows into knowledge, that it involves a conscious choice to change to a healthier lifestyle. Several authors have shown that people transform over time as they learn new skills and techniques to eliminate the barriers to change.[19,20] However, awareness and knowledge, while necessary, will not usually be sufficient to produce recommended changes in risky health behaviors. Nurses often know they should change behaviors—for example, should lose weight, stop smoking, or get more exercise, yet don't often do so. How often has an individual resolved in January to make some change in his or her life, yet made little progress and within eight weeks loses the drive to continue that commitment?

Changing to a healthier lifestyle requires an attitude change, which involves commitment. As one contemplates the changes needed to improve health, the nurse must be constantly reminded to move beyond the physical dimensions of self-care and recognize that well-being, in anyone's life, means whole person care. The nurse must provide for the attentive balance in each aspect of the individual's physical, mental, emotional, social, spiritual, vocational, and environmental health. This awareness is the foundation for change; and while certain choices may seem commonplace, when all aspects of one's being are considered, the change becomes crucial to avoiding the risk of unnecessary illness or premature death.

Table 3–3 illustrates the nursing knowledge and skill required for a nurse to meet Standard 3.1.3.

Table 3–3 Eliminating At-Risk Health Behaviors

Standard of Practice 3.1.3	*Key Concepts*	*Requisite Knowledge*	*Requisite Skills*
Holistic nurses recognize and address at-risk health patterns and begin the process of change.	Eliminating at-risk health patterns.	Understanding concepts of self-awareness and self-knowledge.	Develop a healthy self-outlook; create energy and vitality in life.
	Lifestyle changes.	Knowledge of general theories of behavior; theories of change or transformation.	Develop interpersonal relationship skills; being internally motivated and possessing an attitude and willingness to commit to preset goals; ability to think positively.
	Change process.	Knowledge of concepts related to skills training; support and adoption of lifestyle changes.	Develop skills to devise an individualized plan for lifestyle change; ability to affirm positive outcomes of improved health and wholeness.

Nursing Activities

Nursing actions that demonstrate this Standard include the use of risk appraisal and risk reduction assessments. Also, identification of barriers to healthy behavior such as health beliefs or attitudes must be uncovered before one can make changes. Primary interventions such as education and counseling facilitate positive health practices and determine the readiness for change. The use of self-help groups and social support groups assists individuals to adopt strategies to keep well.

Determining effective planning of individual care requires assessment and evaluation of health attitudes, values, beliefs, health behaviors, and social support systems. Value-consistent health behaviors are necessary to being truly engaged or committed to change to a healthier lifestyle.[3] Often, holistic nurses use the Health Belief Model to guide practice. This theory directs the nurse to focus on assessment of a person's willingness to accept health care advice. Further, this model guides the nurse to focus on how persons perceive their physical impairment, the extent of risk when they take no action, the extent to which this change impacts their social life, and their confidence with the proposed treatment regime.

For holistic nurses, clarifying values and beliefs is perhaps the single most important technique to assist one to achieve a balanced lifestyle. Participating in exercises that involve values clarification methods helps one to recognize those things that are important, meaningful, and valuable in life. Further, these exercises help one to evaluate what behaviors or attitudes need to be changed, particularly those that are not consistent with one's beliefs. Devising an action plan based on realistic, positive goals can lead to success and bring about the needed change.

One more key to successful change is recognizing that motivation, while critically important, is not sufficient to ensure that one will sustain the needed change. Dossey describes a spiral model of the changes one frequently cycles through: the more actions one takes, the greater the success rate over time.[3] Understanding how one moves through the various stages and knowing that relapse is common, nurses are less likely to allude to failure but rather they will encourage others to learn from their mistakes. Studies have also shown that support and encouragement make change last.[21] This requires the use of effective helping relationships, such as those found in self-help groups and social support groups whose primary intent is to encourage the development of new attitudes and behaviors and thus increase the potential to change.[22]

CASE STUDIES

1 Nurse Adele uses the Health Belief Model with her clients and knows that it is essential that she understand her clients' beliefs and values to implement behavioral changes and needed lifestyle modifications. Adele, however, knows that she herself has to lose weight and exercise more. She has never been successful with dieting in the past even though she has joined every weight program in her community.

Yet, this time it seems different. Adele has developed a different philosophy that truly demonstrates taking control over her choices. She has identified a basic plan to eat well using the Food Pyramid as a guide to balanced meal planning. Further, she has set realistic goals for a personal fitness plan and identified ways to overcome barriers that prevented her from adhering to a daily exercise plan in the past. Most important, Adele has learned that relapse is common and she does not view her past experiences as failures; but rather, she has empowered herself to become healthier. Adele has become aware of her own individual lifestyle patterns that had turned into barriers to being healthy. Similarly, Adele guides her clients to eliminate, reduce, or manage those risk behaviors by learning to recognize which cultural beliefs, values, concerns, or practices cause barriers to a healthy lifestyle. Adele meets Standard 3.1.3.

2 Nurse Irene works in a wellness clinic where she counsels consumers, clients, and providers on smoking cessation. Irene recognizes the importance of educating providers and clients about tobacco use and its impact on health. During her education sessions, she hands out pamphlets on the risks of smoking including handouts showing statistics on the morbidity and mortality rates associated with tobacco use. Irene frequently shows audio-visuals that depict the struggles clients face when they suffer from Chronic Obstructive Pulmonary Disease (COPD).

When Irene drives home from work, she does not use a seat belt, believing she is as much at risk from having the seat belt on as not wearing one. Irene's experience relates back to a very good friend who died in a car accident when he was trapped and workers could not release the seat belt. While reports showed her friend died of internal injuries sustained in the accident, Irene believes he may have been saved if workers had gotten him out in time. While Irene's caring interventions in her clinical practice at the wellness clinic do meet this Standard, she has failed to internalize the extent of risk she poses to herself daily by not wearing a seat belt. Irene has not accepted the potential dangers to one's well-being associated with not using seat belts, nor has she accepted the medical reports that indicate the cause of death of her friend.

Standard of Practice 3.1.4

Holistic nurses consciously cultivate awareness and understanding about the deeper meaning, purpose, inner strengths, and connections with self, others, nature, and God/Life Force/Absolute/Transcendent.

This Standard reflects the capacity one has to recognize and assess the wholeness existing within self and others. By consciously cultivating awareness of self, the whole being—including one's physical, mental, emotional, and spiritual natures and one's relationships and choices—has the capacity to change or to take on new meaning, contributing to a greater feeling of self-worth. By coming to know one's self, nurses have a deeper understanding of their mission in life. By nurturing the spirit or caring for the spirit/soul, nurses gain inner strength. By journeying in reflective thought, nurses experience solitude, inspiration, and growth and ultimately gain an ability to live in a healing way, to have a life of loving usefulness. An outcome of knowing one's own inner self can be the ability to guide and nurture the healing of others, to assist others in finding meaning, purpose, love, and hope. This Standard dictates that the holistic nurse understand the meaning of the circle of human potential and value the importance of self-assessments.[3,19,20,23]

Table 3–4 illustrates the nursing knowledge and skill required for a nurse to meet Standard 3.1.4.

Table 3–4 Unfolding the Power within and through Connections

Standard of Practice 3.1.4	*Key Concepts*	*Requisite Knowledge*	*Requisite Skills*
Holistic nurses consciously cultivate awareness and understanding about the deeper meaning, purpose, inner strengths, and connections with self, others, nature, and God/Life Force/Absolute/Transcendent.	Conscious awareness and understanding of self.	Personal, interpersonal, and transpersonal dimensions of self; exploration of perceptions of "meaning."	Self-validation; focusing on what happens within; affirmations of exceptional qualities.
	Interconnectedness with others.	Levels of therapeutic presence; understanding self as a resource to others.	Engage in activities to keep community with others alive and heart-centered; establish and maintain meaningful relationships.
	Interconnectedness with nature.	Levels of human experience; unity and oneness with the environment, the universe.	Engage in activities to protect other life forms and the Earth as a whole.
	Interconnectedness with God/Life Force/Absolute/Transcendent.	Concepts related to spiritual experiences and inner movements of the spirit; concepts related to embodied soul.	Explore beliefs, feelings, meaning, and purpose of life; affirm a relative capacity for faith.

Nursing Activities

Nursing actions that demonstrate this Standard include transpersonal caring and healing awareness, such as nursing assessments, that explore sources of inner strength. Other actions include supporting opportunities for making important connections; providing for activities that nurture, such as respect for meaningful rituals; and providing for activities that promote levels of trust and recognize fear levels.

Transpersonal caring and healing awareness refer to experiences and meanings that go beyond individual uniqueness; they involve purpose, meaning, and values.[3] By encouraging individuals to develop a deeper sense of purpose in life and to become connected with their own spiritual being, nurses learn to facilitate a more harmonious interconnection with and between others, with their physical environments and with God/Life Force/Absolute/Transcendent. When practice is consistent with the role of healer, nurses allow others to be who they are, avoiding the need to control, to judge another, or to change another in a way that is incongruent with their own personal values and beliefs.[23] By creating healing environments, the nurse can demonstrate his or her healing power by being fully with another through listening with their whole being—by pausing, taking time, and paying attention. In such healing situations, nurses assist others to bring all parts of their being into a deeper level of inner knowing, leading to integration and balance.[24]

Healing environments can be created when nurses demonstrate ability to listen and to remain centered. Listening actively and with intention allows nurses the opportunity to teach clients to reframe experiences positively. In so doing, they guide clients to increase inner awareness, improve self-understanding, and ultimately recognize one's human potential to heal. Further, interventions should also include the use of a variety of appropriate caring methods for healing, such as prayer, grief support groups, reminiscence therapy, use of clergy, and advocating one's position when one's religious beliefs conflict with routine medical regimes. In some situations, the use of prayer and religious reading material can be as important as facilitating one's participation in religious ritual or protection of one's religious articles.[7,8,9]

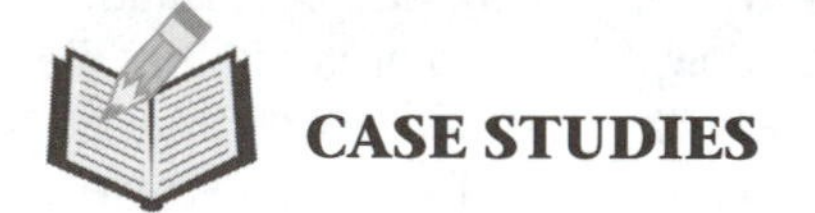

CASE STUDIES

1 Nurse Alayna was caring for Aaron, a client with AIDS who had been admitted to the hospital with a variety of symptoms associated with his illness (daily fevers, weight loss, skin rashes, psychomotor retardation, withdrawal, lethargy, and inability to respond to loved ones). Aaron feared the illness and was very afraid of death. He had, up until now, totally avoided discussing the issues surrounding his diagnosis. His wife reported that he had been experiencing severe depression and had been unable to work. He had also dropped out of the therapy sessions with his counselor. During this hospitalization, Nurse Alayna discussed fear with Aaron and openly examined her own apprehensions, remaining centered, aware of emotions, and nonjudgmental. Aaron began to deal with his self-blame. He had extremes of self-deprecation alternating with further periods of despairing of ever recovering. The discussions between Nurse Alayna and Aaron centered on the emotional distress of his life-threatening condition, as well as the mental anguish and guilt, the financial drain his illness was imposing on his family, and the spiritual questioning that led to identifying his relationship with his God.

By remaining compassionate in all interactions, Nurse Alayna disclosed information that validated for Aaron that both he and Nurse Alayna had formed a trusting connection. They had created an authentic relationship and had come together as a "whole." For Aaron, these encounters created a healing awareness. Aaron felt not only that he was a part of the care provided by Nurse Alayna but also that he was worthy of care. He felt that he was being loved unconditionally.

Nurse Alayna met Standard 3.1.4 because her caring attitude allowed a transpersonal perspective to emerge where the whole self of the nurse is brought into relationship with the whole self of the client. Nurse Alayna offered herself in a healing relationship, meeting Aaron where he was with his illness without judgment and offering healing in love.

2 Micah was a nurse working with AIDS clients in a large acute care setting in the Northeast. He enjoyed his work, finding the clients' physical, emotional, and social conditions challenging. Micah also enjoyed working with his coworkers and colleagues, but feared they would discover that he also led a life that exposed him to this disease that has no known cure. In trying to hide his vulnerability and recent diagnosis that he is infected with HIV, Micah became less able to be compassionate and began to voice prejudicial comments. He questioned his own future: Will my pain be manageable, will my loved ones be with me, will my colleagues still respect me, is there life after death? Why me? Why this illness and all of its life-threatening dimensions? Micah did not meet Standard 3.1.4 because he was unable to overcome his own personal pain and tend to the needs of others with compassion.

Standard of Practice 3.1.5

Holistic nurses use clear intention to care for self and to seek a sense of balance, harmony, and joy in daily life.

This Standard focuses on the nurse as a person who clearly uses holistic nursing intervention strategies and modalities for himself/herself. Using self-care strategies on one's own behalf to maintain wholeness and well-being is paramount to increasing levels of contentment, comfort, and peace of mind. For example, in the process of caring for self, nurses frequently use humor and laughter as a healing strategy to relieve stress.[17] Equally important, however, nurses use healing techniques to understand who they are as a person and why they have come to be the person they are. Nurses think of their life as a tapestry woven into an intricate pattern that highlights important aspects of their being. Self-reflection can be a transformational process whereby nurses become aware of themselves as new beings; self-empowered, self-fulfilled, and eager to advocate and be connected to others. From the perspective of their professional practice, once nurses participate in self-reflection activities, they gain a deeper understanding of the meaning and essence of caring for people.[19,20]

Table 3–5 illustrates the nursing knowledge and skill required for a nurse to meet Standard 3.1.5.

Table 3–5 Caring Responsibly for Self

Standard of Practice 3.1.5	*Key Concepts*	*Requisite Knowledge*	*Requisite Skills*
Holistic nurses use clear intention to care for self and to seek a sense of balance, harmony, and joy in daily life.	Consciously designing ways to maximize one's potential.	Knowledge of body-mind connections; concepts of health and wellness and related risks.	Plan self-care activities to promote health and prevent disease; activities to maintain a sense of balance.
	Living a balanced, harmonious, and joyful daily life.	Human response patterns; concepts related to the importance and interdependence of all segments of individual being—physical, mental, emotional, spiritual, and relationships, and choices.	Use of alternative therapies and/or relaxation interventions to promote wellness behaviors; discovering the authentic, satisfying, fulfilling joys and pleasures of human life.

Nursing Activities

Nursing actions that demonstrate this Standard include: holistic self-health and stress assessments; daily journaling; exploring and using relaxation strategies, such as visualization, and coping strategies, such as healthy nutrition and exercise.

Holistic self-health and stress assessments are the processes used to access one's own inner wisdom. It is listening to one's own story about self to discover not only the unity of one's body and mind but also one's interrelatedness with others and the whole universe.[3] Holistic health assessment is learning about one's lifestyle and the habits that contribute to wellness or impose constraints on health and well-being. By using self-health, lifestyle, or stress assessments, one learns of the health-enhancing changes needed to maintain or restore oneself to a healthier state of being that increases the ability to resist disease.

Journaling is commonly used in nursing, particularly in mental health settings, as a way to keep a record of personal thoughts, experiences, and reactions to events. However, journaling is also an excellent self-care strategy to record one's subjective interpretations and goals for lifestyle changes. Like a diary, one's journal record is private correspondence seldom, if ever, shared with another and an extremely helpful way to gain awareness of one's personal values.

Imagery is a process used to assist one to journey inward to experience personal memories, dreams, fantasies, and visions. It serves as a bridge for connecting a person's body-mind-spirit, and usually the process involves one or more of the senses. Imagery is an extremely helpful way to assist individuals in the healing process.[3,25]

Learning to be responsible to self requires motivation and commitment along with goal setting and the use of strategies such as frequent self-reflection, self-monitoring, setting aside expectations, and allowing humor and joyful living to enter into one's personal world.

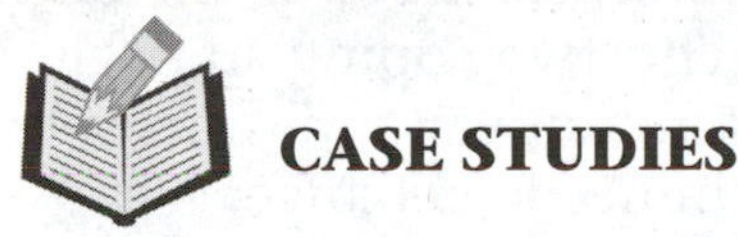

CASE STUDIES

1 Belinda is a nurse who does morning breath work daily. She acknowledges every day as a new beginning; she takes three deep breaths and thanks God for her life. As a hospice nurse, Belinda works with the dying. She frequently has stressful days but avoids becoming overwhelmed because she interacts with her clients by consistently offering a caring presence, comfort, and loving connections. She takes a deep breath and really listens as her clients talk about their pain, knowing that the listening is the loving. Belinda uses her breath work throughout the day to relieve stress and bring about an inner calm. After work hours, Belinda allows her inner self to experience humor and joyful moments. She enjoys her many relationships, knowing her family and friends are the essence of her life, which allows her the opportunity to love and be loved. Belinda meets Standard 3.1.5 because she values her well-being and believes that it contributes to the quality of care offered to her clients.

2 Abigail, a nurse clinician diagnosed with systemic lupus, took great pride in the fact that she created a daily ritual for herself to deal with the many emotional stresses in her life brought about by her physical ailments. Abigail was newly married and wanted to have a child but was cautioned that a pregnancy could worsen her physical condition. Since she had always followed a healthy lifestyle, Abigail was unclear as to why she had to face this consequence of an incurable illness, though her faith in God was never shaken. She created a sacred space to be alone, to meditate and reflect, consistently deepening her understanding of being connected with self, others, and God. Abigail knew this healing ritual reduced her anxiety and fear of an uncertain future; it lessened her feelings of helplessness that sometimes occurred because of her frequent joint pains or her feelings of despair at not being able to give birth to her own child. Abigail used the health-enhancing technique of meditation to refresh her body-mind-spirit connection. Abigail met Standard 3.1.5 because she created a healing awareness to restore herself to a healthier state of being and she was more able to resist the disease.

Standard of Practice 3.1.6

Holistic nurses participate in the evolutionary holistic process with the understanding that crisis creates opportunity in any setting.

This Standard emphasizes the importance of meaning and wholeness and the art of helping relationships. One of the few constants in life is knowing that change in response to life events occurs daily. How individuals react to a life event that causes stress can affect their well-being. In situations that are less threatening, individuals adapt using similar coping strategies as in previous responses to stress. However, when the stress is perceived as a crisis, the individual's usual coping patterns are weakened or they fall apart. Life events that require major changes can become an opportunity to learn new, more adaptive ways to handle one's life. It provides an opportunity to expand one's awareness and potential. This Standard dictates that nurses offer the clients support and validations to help them to identify effective coping strategies to correct distortions. By helping clients to clarify and understand, nurses help them to experience self-discovery and participate in needed change.

Table 3–6 illustrates the nursing knowledge and skill required for a nurse to meet Standard 3.1.6.

Table 3–6 Growing through Crisis

Standard of Practice 3.1.6	*Key Concepts*	*Requisite Knowledge*	*Requisite Skills*
Holistic nurses participate in the evolutionary holistic process with the understanding that crisis creates opportunity in any setting.	Evolutionary holistic process.	Theories of change, natural adaptation, and knowing the meaning of having a purpose in life; theories of communication.	Therapeutic helping skills; finding an effective, appropriate, and lasting source of motivation; understanding and using therapeutic communication skills effectively.
	Using crisis as a basis to create opportunity.	Concepts related to maintaining hope, continuity, and connectedness to life.	Coping strategies; accepting responsibility for freedom of self-determination.

Nursing Activities

Nursing actions that demonstrate this Standard include: therapeutic communication and basic counseling approaches; healing interventions that focus on the feelings, needs, problems, and challenges that one faces in times of crisis; supporting clients in becoming assertive and accepting responsibility for self-discovery of their own healing power.

Therapeutic communication techniques used in crisis and post-crisis situations are purposefully intended to assist one to learn how one responds to a serious problem, hence leading to well-being and more positive responses. Basic counseling involves establishing relationships that focus on relieving mental and emotional stress and result in acceptance, authenticity, and empathy. To facilitate communication with the client, the nurse should use helping skills such as active listening or primary-level empathy. Further, the nurse should encourage dialogue that allows the client to hear himself or herself, since this engages individuals in active problem solving, leads them to a new understanding of what is truly important in life, and guides them to deal with crisis in a positive way.[10] Thus, in crisis situations, the goal is to assist clients to reflect and to express feelings, including clarifying and interpreting to provide information and feedback, to select and weigh alternatives, and to develop a spiritual understanding about one's life. Ultimately, the longer-range goal is to motivate clients to work toward their life's potential.

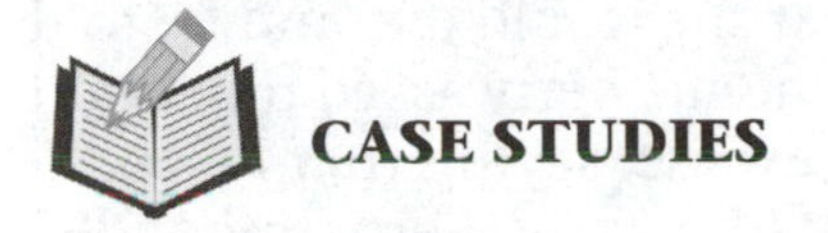

CASE STUDIES

1 Louise, an emergency room clinical specialist, worked at Valley Regional Medical Center. She had been married to Travis, a bank vice-president, for 35 years. Their life together had been happy until Travis's recent job loss when his bank merged with a larger company and the reorganization eliminated his position. He seemed to be coping with this loss, but Louise had noticed he looked more withdrawn lately and uninterested in any family activity. Louise, carrying the burden as sole provider, would easily lose patience with him. Her colleagues often heard her on the phone lecturing Travis, saying, "You are not the only 55-year-old who has ever lost a job."

One afternoon, an ambulance arrived at the emergency department (ED), and Louise noticed that one of her sons was following close behind the stretcher. Louise panicked and had to be quieted and brought to another room by Sylvia as emergency personnel worked to revive her husband. Louise was in shock and unable to forgive herself for being angry with Travis. Now that his life was in jeopardy because he had overdosed on his medications, she feared she would not be able to tell him how much she really did love him.

Louise's immediate supervisor, Sylvia, the ED nurse manager, was extremely helpful and supportive in guiding Louise by listening to Louise as she conveyed how important her husband was to her in her life and by communicating with her quietly. Yet Sylvia provided specific directions on what Louise needed to do to help her husband during this immediate crisis. She encouraged Louise and her son to contact other family members, and she gently talked to them about the approach they would need to have in their first communications with Travis. Sylvia reminded Louise of how well she advocated for clients when they were in similar situations. She highlighted Louise's strengths and reminded her of how often she discussed, with her clients, the importance of prayer in the healing process. Sylvia also reminded Louise of how confident she was in dealing with crises in the work setting and supported her by saying how she believed she could also do this in dealing with a crisis in her own life.

Sylvia, the nurse manager, met Standard 3.1.6 because she maintained a calm controlled presence. She was nonjudgmental of Louise's behavioral responses to crisis situations in her own life. Rather, she linked the emotional responses that Louise had been having for days to the past crisis of her husband's job loss and not to insensitivity toward another person's problems. She engaged Louise in problem solving, and she offered reassuring support. She helped Louise to regain a sense of hope that soon their family life would once again be functional.

2 Ramon, a 64-year-old male, was sitting outside the Intensive Care Unit while his wife lay dying from complications associated with the advanced stages of COPD. When Kerry, his wife's nurse, invited him into the unit to see his wife, he refused, saying he wanted to let her rest. Ramon clearly believed she needed all her energy to recover. Even though he had been told of the seriousness of his wife's condition, he was denying that she would die, and he told Kerry of the arrangements he had made to take her home. Kerry asked him again to visit his wife and he responded with a second excuse, saying that he could not be cheerful and he did not want his wife to see him upset. Kerry responded by saying, "I'll tell your wife you have gone to the cafeteria for dinner."

Rather than listening to the content of what Ramon was saying or to the feelings he was expressing, Kerry abandoned Ramon at a time of great need. Kerry did not meet Standard 3.1.6 because she did not intervene in a therapeutic way, nor did she assist Ramon to identify coping strategies or develop viable solutions to his existing crisis.

CONCLUSION

Core Value 3 reflects on the standards of holistic nursing practice that support the self-care approach to lifestyle change. These standards emphasize the strong belief that nurses must first take care of themselves before they are able to deliver transformational care to their clients. Ultimately, holistic nurses have the responsibility to model health behaviors, to achieve harmony and balance in their own lives, and to assist others striving to do the same.

In addition, Core Value 3 describes self-care as consisting of the self-initiated activities directed toward maintaining life, health, and well-being. Fundamental to ensuring achievement of these goals is the philosophy of mind/body/spirit connections and their ability to influence the healing experience. Yet, before nurses are able to facilitate the healing in others, they must, by being consciously aware, acknowledge and nurture their own healer within.

At-risk behaviors, in Core Value 3, are viewed as barriers that may interfere with successfully achieving lifestyle change. However, barriers are merely obstacles that can be identified and overcome by adopting innovative approaches such as self-monitoring, goal setting, and interventions aimed at health promotion—for example, establishing an exercise regime, participating in stress management activities, or using positive reaffirmations. Other requisite skills include developing a clear intention to live a balanced life, to allow humor and joy to be part of one's daily routines. Using image visualization to change behavior or seeking social support from others is helpful to many. Still others find solace by developing a belief or faith in a higher power or connecting with nature and experiencing a unity and oneness with the environment and the universe. Crisis is viewed as opportunity in any setting where the nurse's focus is to assist in reducing and controlling risks to health while strengthening positive health behaviors.

NOTES

1. R.S. Ryan and J.W. Travis, *Wellness: Small Changes You Can Make To Make a Big Difference* (Berkeley, CA: Ten Speed Press, 1991).
2. P.C. Foster and N.P. Janssens, "Dorothea E. Orem," in *Nursing Theories: The Basis for Professional Nursing Practice*, 2d ed., eds. N.T.C. Group (Englewood Cliffs, NJ: Prentice-Hall, 1980), 124–139.
3. B.M. Dossey et al., *Holistic Nursing: A Handbook for Practice*, 3d ed. (Gaithersburg, MD: Aspen Publishers, 2000).
4. M.J. McKivergin and M.J. Daubenmire, "The Healing Process of Presence," *Journal of Holistic Nursing* 12, no. 1 (1994): 65–81.
5. M.J. McKivergen, "The Nurse As an Instrument of Healing," in *American Holistic Nurses' Association Core Curriculum for Holistic Nursing*, ed. B.M. Dossey (Gaithersburg, MD: Aspen Publishers, 1997).
6. J. Campbell and M. Kreidler, "Older Adults' Perceptions about Wellness," *Journal of Holistic Nursing* 12, no. 4 (1994): 437–447.
7. D.A. Matthews, *The Faith Factor* (New York, Viking Press, 1998).
8. T.E. Oxman et al., "Lack of Social Participation or Religious Strength or Comfort As Risk Factors for Death after Cardiac Surgery in the Elderly," *Psychosomatic Medicine* 57 (1995): 5–15.
9. W.J. Strawbridge et al., "Frequent Attendance at Religious Services and Mortality over 28 Years," *American Journal of Public Health* 87 (1997): 957–961.
10. E. Arnold and K.U. Boggs, *Interpersonal Relationships*, 3d ed. (Philadelphia: W.B. Saunders, 1999).
11. M.G. Rubenfeld and B.K. Scheffer, *Critical Thinking in Nursing: An Interactive Approach*, 2d ed. (Philadelphia: J.B. Lippincott Co., 1999).
12. M.A. Burkhardt and A.K. Nathaniel, *Ethics & Issues in Contemporary Nursing* (Albany, NY: Delmar Publishers, 1998).
13. B.A. Hall, "Spirituality in Terminal Illness: An Alternative View of Theory," *Journal of Holistic Nursing* 15, no. 1 (1997): 82–95.
14. M.L. Kendall, "A Holistic Nursing Model for Spiritual Care of the Terminally Ill," *American Journal of Hospice & Palliative Care* 16, no. 2 (1999): 473–476.
15. G.M. Timmerman, "Using Self-Care Strategies To Make Lifestyle Changes," *Journal of Holistic Nursing* 17, no. 2 (1999): 169–183.
16. C.E. Guzzetta, ed., *Essential Readings in Holistic Nursing* (Gaithersburg, MD: Aspen Publishers, 1998), 95.
17. P. Wooten, "Humor: An Antidote for Stress," in *Essential Readings in Holistic Nursing*, ed. C.E. Guzzetta (Gaithersburg, MD: Aspen Publishers, 1998), 133–139.
18. J. Walton, "Spirituality of Patients Recovering from an Acute Myocardial Infarction," *Journal of Holistic Nursing* 17, no. 1 (1999): 34–53.

19. S.S. Lauterbach and P.H. Becker, "Caring for Self: Becoming a Self-Reflective Nurse," in *Essential Readings in Holistic Nursing*, ed. C.E. Guzzetta (Gaithersburg, MD: Aspen Publishers, 1998), 97–107.
20. C.L. Wells-Federman, "Awakening the Nurse Healer Within," in *Essential Readings in Holistic Nursing*, ed. C.E. Guzzetta (Gaithersburg, MD: Aspen Publishers, 1998), 108–122.
21. J. Campbell and M. Kreidler, "Older Adults' Perceptions about Wellness," *Journal of Holistic Nursing* 17, no. 3 (1999): 437–447.
22. C.A. Baer, "Smoking Assessment and Intervention: An Essential Part of Disease Treatment," in *Essential Readings in Holistic Nursing*, ed. C.E. Guzzetta (Gaithersburg, MD: Aspen Publishers, 1998), 197–205.
23. L. Keegan, *The Nurse As Healer* (Albany, NY: Delmar Publishers, 1994).
24. M.E. Doona et al., "Nursing Presence: As Real As a Milky Way Bar," *Journal of Holistic Nursing* 17, no. 1 (1999): 54–70.
25. B.M. Dossey, *American Holistic Nurses' Association Core Curriculum for Holistic Nursing* (Gaithersburg, MD: Aspen Publishers, 1997), 188–195.

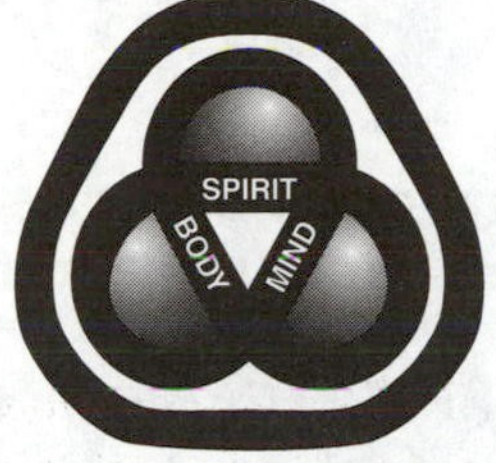

CORE VALUE 4

HOLISTIC COMMUNICATION, THERAPEUTIC ENVIRONMENT, AND CULTURAL DIVERSITY

Johanne A. Quinn

4.1 Holistic Communication

Holistic nurses engage in holistic communication to ensure that each person experiences the presence of the nurse as authentic and sincere; there is an atmosphere of shared humanness that includes a sense of connectedness and attention reflecting the individual's uniqueness.

Communication is the primary method used to establish and maintain the nurse-client relationship. It is a Core Value in the practice of holistic nursing and an essential activity in the caring for and healing of clients. For holistic communication to be effective, the nurse must understand the concepts of sender (the source or initiator of a message), message (the verbal and nonverbal behaviors conveyed through words, gestures, expressions, and behaviors), and receiver (the interpreter who decodes the message and gives meaning to the message). Further, in communicating with clients, the nurse must demonstrate the ability to integrate core helping skills such as empathy, respect, genuine concern, understanding, and willingness to listen in the process of developing a level of trust with the client. Clearly, to comprehend what the client is saying, the nurse must be silent. The nurse must listen actively with intention so that the interchange occurs within an atmosphere of shared humanness. According to Dossey, to listen with intention, the nurse quiets his or her inner thoughts and is present in the moment, listening quietly and avoiding preconceived ideas or attempts to analyze what one thinks the other means.[1]

An inherently important goal in all nurse-client interactions is to ensure that nurses take into account the necessary "therapeutic" communication skills, thus creating a rewarding exchange of information. Accordingly, for holistic communication to be effective, nurses and clients must share an experience of valued interchange (authenticity) in which facts, feelings, and meanings are exchanged. The client must receive the message exactly as the nurse intended it to be. Likewise, when the client sends his or her message, the nurse must receive the message as intended. Each person must be continually aware of the other, adapting and adjusting as necessary, so that a genuine connectedness occurs between the nurse and the client. For the nurse, it requires gathering information by listening, perceiving, attaching meaning, and prioritizing a relative importance to interactions. Clients may respond to an interaction based on past experience or even perceptions developed as a result of awareness and the excitation of the senses, all of which can have a profound effect on the communication process.

The Standards on holistic communication are equally important concepts to put into practice within the realm of daily interactions with others. For instance, in the work setting, maintaining eye contact, keeping promises, showing empathy, maintaining an open communication style, listening attentively, and intentionally, and using clarification for things not understood are clearly effective tools in communicating. By way of illustration, nurses must maintain effective communication skills in conversations and in listening with colleagues, peers, coworkers, physicians, or those in authority such as supervisors, managers, or administrators. Thus, particularly effective approaches with these individuals would be to use "I" messages. As an example, nurses often work in situations where they must deal with conflict, mistrust, and disrespect. In such instances, the goal for communication by the sender (the nurse) would be to avoid creating a defensive reaction on the part of the receiver (the physician). Nurses must learn how to use disarming language over arming language. The more hostile communication is, the less accurately it may be heard. Consequently, an important sending skill for the nurse is to make a point and express emotions through "I" messages. This technique often works to expand an opponent's ability to listen and hear. Such messages locate the conflict outside of the listener, where reframing can be more easily accomplished to bring about a cooperative, more collegial resolution. "I" messages also focus on behavior rather than person as the source of the conflict and are less likely to be felt as personal attacks. "I" messages encourage a similar "I" response from the "other."

Standard of Practice 4.1.1

Holistic nurses develop an awareness of the most frequently encountered challenges to holistic communication.

This Standard calls attention to the importance of developing the art of "listening" as a technique to enhance communicating with clients. It is the basis of all interpersonal relationships to ensure that nurses and clients understand each other. By involving themselves in what the client is saying, nurses become genuine listeners and avoid interrupting or jumping to conclusions. Furthermore, nurses who are good listeners avoid advising; they become "good listeners" without being selective about what they expect to hear. Asking questions to clarify without presuming they understood what the speaker means is also an excellent technique to keep communication alive. By using effective patterns of communication, the nurse encourages and supports self-discovery on the part of the client.[2] Realizing that communication can take a long time to process, it becomes critical to display an unhurried manner and to allow the interchange to occur when the client is ready and on the client's own terms. Quite honestly, it soon becomes easy to hear a person's soft voice or even to understand the meaning of a clenched fist without becoming judgmental or attempting to force communication by saying, "I see your fist is clenched—can you tell me why you are angry?"

Table 4–1 illustrates the nursing knowledge and skill required for a nurse to meet Standard 4.1.1.

Table 4–1 Challenges to Holistic Communication

Standard of Practice 4.1.1	*Key Concepts*	*Requisite Knowledge*	*Requisite Skills*
Holistic nurses develop an awareness of the most frequently encountered challenges to holistic communication.	Holistic communication.	Basic concepts of communication; therapeutic communication process; intuitive knowing and energetic vibrations.	Relationship skills; core helping skills; focused exploration and problem-solving skills.
	Discerning challenges in communication.	Concepts related to perceptions; self-beliefs; perceived threats; pain; crisis; and interpersonal communication.	Recognizing barriers to communication during the assessment, intervention, evaluation phase of the nursing process and in written communication.

Nursing Activities

Nursing actions that demonstrate this Standard include: developing professional communication skills, using core helping skills, creating opportunities for focused explorations, and using active problem-solving strategies.

Developing professional communication skills, the basic tool of all helping relationships, requires the nurse to establish positive rapport with clients including the effective use of listening skills, use of verbal and nonverbal techniques, and effective written communication skills. The effective use of core helping skills involves the ability to demonstrate qualities of empathy, respect, and genuineness. Since positive therapeutic relationships are core to providing holistic care, the guiding principle must then convey to the client that he or she is being understood, that what he or she is saying is accurate and the right choice at this time in his or her life. Additionally, when the goal is to establish a therapeutic relationship, nurses must assist the client to clarify the meaning of events. This can happen by asking a question that focuses on how, what, when, where, or under what circumstances.[2] The use of core helping skills is also essential to the healing process; they are aimed at purposeful sharing through focused exploration leading to self-discovery for the client. The client will attest to feelings of being heard and understood as opposed to misinterpretation of meaning (what the client knows, wants, and needs for himself or herself). Techniques to help one with self-discovery may include such activities as journaling, art therapy, letter writing, or reinforcing personal strengths and resources. By using these skills effectively, nurses assist clients to actively problem-solve and gain an even deeper meaning of their behavior, thus resulting in a human connectedness between the nurse and the client.[2]

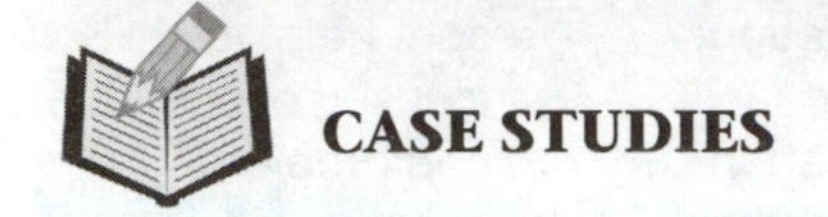

CASE STUDIES

1 Nurse Natasha, an oncology nurse specialist, is caring for Roseanne, who recently underwent a bone marrow transplant. Natasha has known Roseanne from previous hospital admissions for the treatment of her leukemia. While Natasha is preparing to administer her medications, Roseanne calls out, "Why do I have to suffer like this?" Natasha responds to Roseanne by setting aside the medications and sitting alongside her, taking her hand. She first clarifies with Roseanne to see if she has pain or new fears and worries not yet expressed. Roseanne looks at Natasha but says nothing. Within a few seconds, they both can be heard saying a prayer asking for strength to endure yet another health challenge. At the end of the prayer, Natasha takes time to remind Roseanne of her strength and past abilities to cope with her illness. She encourages Roseanne to stay close to her family and friends who were a great source of support in the past.

Natasha meets Standard 4.1.1 in several ways. First, she successfully developed a positive relationship demonstrating empathy, respect, and genuineness. Additionally, Natasha avoided setting up barriers to communication by continuing to administer the medication and paying no attention to Roseanne's call for understanding. Further, she avoided prejudging Roseanne's feelings or suggesting she should be thankful for so many other things in life. Natasha recognized the importance of being in the moment with Roseanne, of listening intently and recognizing Roseanne's need for prayer.

2 Nurse Briana works at the Morris Rehabilitation Center on a head trauma unit. Willie, her client for the past several weeks, is being treated for severe head trauma as the result of a serious motorcycle accident. Willie's future has been dramatically changed; at 22 years of age, he is now a quadriplegic with severe cognitive dysfunction. Willie's parents visit daily. They are preparing to take him home but confide in Briana that they are fearful because of his frequent outbursts of yelling and his total dependency needs for personal care. Willie's parents say to Briana, "You have such patience with Willie and you ask him what he needs and wants even though he is unable to answer you in an intelligent way. He does things for you but we fear he will not do anything for us once we get him home. What should we do?"

Briana pauses for a few minutes and then shares with Willie's parents that she did not always have the patience to handle a person with major disabilities. She shares that she always completed tasks for them because it helped her to get her work done on time. However, as she reflected on who she had become as a nurse, she was saddened that she had lost sight of treating her clients as "whole beings" deserving of care and respect. Now Briana approaches her daily responsibilities by offering quality care that will not only foster more independence but will also assist individuals to achieve their maximum potential. Continuing in conversation with Willie's parents, Briana says, "People like your son Willie re-learn to do so much for themselves and they are so proud of their accomplishments. Do you think you could learn to be patient with Willie in the same way? Could you talk to him each day and wait for him to give some sort of an answer? Can you help him to feed himself with his adaptive spoon?"

Briana meets Standard 4.1.1 because she adapts her communication methods appropriately for her disabled clients. Her communication methods with Willie's parents showed an insightful reflection, and she shared a part of her professional self with them in an attempt to lead them into deeper self-exploration of their abilities to care for their disabled son.

3 Margaret, a school nurse, is preparing to teach a health education class to unwed teenagers who are pregnant for the second time. The information she plans to share has been collected from the local health department; it is relevant information on self care—the discomforts of pregnancy, caring for the newborn, sibling response to a new baby, caring for children as a single parent, and contraceptive use following delivery of a newborn. When it comes time to share this information, Margaret does not discuss any of the issues with the girls individually. Rather, she begins her presentation by lecturing on the problems teenage mothers face with two children and the difficulties they will encounter in completing their high school education. She also addressed the cost of day care and the need to locate reliable baby sitters. Margaret talks about medical expenses and, in particular, the young girls' need to consider a contraceptive method such as tubal ligation.

Margaret fails to meet Standard 4.1.1 since she does not treat the young teenage girls with respect, she fails to individualize their teaching needs, and she assumes their recidivism will continue by suggesting a permanent method of birth control. Margaret has set up many barriers to establishing a nurse-client relationship; she fails to maintain positive communication interactions during her teaching sessions with these young girls. Her presentation style is confrontational and accusatory rather than an attempt to bring about a more focused exploration to help the young girls to problem-solve. Margaret's presentation style assumes that all the teenage girls have similar home situations and health care needs.

Standard of Practice 4.1.2

Holistic nurses increase therapeutic and cultural competence skills to enhance their effectiveness through listening to themselves and others.

This Standard accents the importance of integrating culturally competent skills into nursing practice by suggesting that nurses develop an awareness of and a sensitivity to people who hold beliefs and values that are different than their own. Nurses develop culturally competent skills by first learning about their own self and listening to what they believe about another's culture. This self-awareness assists the nurse to recognize that his or her beliefs and behaviors are not common to all. Further, nurses learn of the uniqueness of another person's cultural norms and values through attentive listening. Since the society we live in is unquestionably diverse, it is important to learn about the different ideals, values, and beliefs of culturally different populations, particularly as such matters affect health care practices. This knowledge can also help bring understanding of the social identity or ethnic origins of groups, especially as related to language or the influence of religion on behaviors and practices.

Table 4–2 illustrates the nursing knowledge and skill required for a nurse to meet Standard 4.1.2.

Table 4–2 Communication for Compassionate Caring Practice

Standard of Practice 4.1.2	*Key Concepts*	*Requisite Knowledge*	*Requisite Skills*
Holistic nurses increase therapeutic and cultural competence skills to enhance their effectiveness through listening to themselves and others.	Therapeutic communication and cultural competence skills.	Professional relationships and healing/caring interventions.	Moral and cultural value orientations; knowledge of self and knowledge of others; communication skills; listening skills.
	Compassionate caring practice.	Nursing knowledge, holistic nursing theories, expertise and intuition skills related to whole-person care; knowledge of client's cultural beliefs, values, and practices.	Use of holistic nursing process; use of "doing" and "being" therapies.

Nursing Activities

Nursing actions that demonstrate this Standard include: use of the holistic nursing process that incorporates concepts of cultural health care assessment; healing/caring interventions that respect and support cultural rituals; and interacting and intervening in a culturally consistent manner.

Interacting and intervening in a culturally consistent manner reflect the ability to facilitate communication and deliver culturally competent care. The client's adherence to a treatment regime and the outcome within the healing process is greatly impacted by the presence or absence of the nurse's ability to understand and accept the cultural beliefs, values, and norms of the client under his or her care. Thus it is essential to recognize that the care of diverse populations is enhanced by knowledge and sensitivity to such variables as age, gender, race, religion, socioeconomic status, and lifestyle choice. Likewise, by understanding cultural concepts, the nurse is in a key position to influence the outcomes of care because nurses can empower an individual to be responsible for his or her own health care needs.

A critical component of providing culturally competent care is ensuring the use of the holistic nursing process that builds the concept of culture into every phase of the process.[3] Thus, cultural areas essential in the assessment phase must focus on sociodemographic and spiritual data as well as particular lifestyle habits surrounding nutrition, exercise, health, and healing practices. Cognitive abilities, decision-making abilities, and the influence of family or religion are all primary considerations in planning interventions. Critical within this phase is the need to identify communication patterns, particularly as they would influence relationships with health care professionals who are often perceived as authority figures. Planning interventions must incorporate cultural healing practices to facilitate compliance.[4] In the evaluation phase, revisions to the care plan should not be made unless the client and any family member who greatly influences the client's decisions are consulted with respect to the effectiveness of the interventions and the acceptability of the outcomes of that care.

CASE STUDIES

1 Rhonda, a public health nurse, was recently assigned to a Mexican-American neighborhood clinic in the downtown section of a major city. This was her first experience in a clinic with clients whose cultural background is different than hers. She took some time to sit quietly and reflect on positive experiences so far. For example, just last week she attended a marriage in which the ritual of a lasso around the man's and woman's necks symbolized their bonding and ensured faithfulness to one another. She marveled at the Mexican-American community's closeness and strong religious beliefs.

During the assessment interview for her first client, Rhonda learned that Miranda believed her illness is the result of witchcraft. She is asking for a *curandero* (a folk practitioner) to treat her. Rhonda told her client that the only safe care she could receive was to follow the directions given to her, particularly since this was a reportable illness and follow-up care through the health department was crucial. Following Miranda's physical exam, Rhonda saw to it that she received a prescription with directions on how to use the medication. Rhonda scheduled a follow-up visit for Miranda, who then went home without giving Rhonda a firm commitment to return.

At the end of the day, Rhonda reflected on what her day had been like and her interactions with Miranda. Rhonda said to her supervisor, "I always thought of myself as being open and flexible and reasonably nonjudgmental, but I found myself acting in a way that was not like me. When caring for Miranda, I realized that, without knowing, I made value judgments. These judgments reflected my inability to accept that others want to handle their illness differently, and their perspectives are equally as important as mine." While Rhonda may have failed to recognize the importance of cultural influence in relation to the care for Miranda, she did deliver appropriate care for a person with an infectious disease. Rhonda meets this Standard because she was able to recognize her shortcomings and she identified for her supervisor how she was going to go about getting the skills necessary to be more culturally sensitive in the future.

2 Josephine, a 93-year-old Canadian woman, has been living in the state of Massachusetts since the age of 13. Since the death of her husband and her mother, she has lived alone in a single-bedroom condominium home on the second floor. She is now hospitalized in a rehabilitation center with a broken wrist and head lacerations as the result of a serious fall in her home. Her son, who is in his sixties, is unable to care for his mother in his home since he is still working and unable to provide for his mother's daily personal needs. Josephine is adamant, however, that she not be placed in a nursing home—to her, that would mean her death is imminent. Josephine took care of her own mother in her home; her mother had lived until the age of 91. All members of her family had cared for their parents, and she expected this would happen for her as well.

The multidisciplinary team at the rehabilitation center is recommending a nursing home based on Josephine's age and instability in walking. Nurse Celeste, recognizing Josephine's strong belief that a nursing home means "the place you go to die," requests that a meeting with Josephine's son be arranged to talk about assisted living arrangements. Celeste is aware of a new facility in town that is run by the Sisters of Providence, and she believes the home environment there and the care by individuals who are of the same religious orientation as Josephine might be a good alternative and a more acceptable solution for Josephine. Celeste documented how Josephine's strength had improved since she was in the rehabilitation center, noting that she is now eating three meals per day. Celeste also noted that Josephine had problems with her knee buckling that possibly contributed to her fall. Her documentation showed that prior to her fall, Josephine had not been wearing her knee brace because it no longer fit properly due to a loss of weight. Celeste also commented on the importance of arranging a site visit to the assisted living facility for Josephine and her son, knowing that once they saw the home and talked to the sisters, an acceptable plan might be arranged.

Two weeks after this team meeting, Josephine was transferred to the assisted living facility accompanied by Celeste and her son. Her eyes were bright with excitement as she walked around her new living room. She said to her son, "I can attend Mass daily. Have you seen the lovely chapel at the end of the hall?"

Celeste meets Standard 4.1.2 because she was sensitive to a 93-year-old woman's need to be cared for in a homelike environment and she took the time to ensure that visits to the home were made prior to arranging for Josephine's transfer. Further, Celeste's documentation on Josephine's particular health-related problems (her weakness from not eating correctly at home and the improperly fitting knee brace) resulted in Josephine being evaluated as a good candidate for admission to an assisted living home.

3 Lucia, a nurse practitioner, is working in a woman's health clinic. Her client is a 42-year-old Hispanic woman recently diagnosed with breast cancer. Lucia is explaining the most common treatment options and the continued care necessary. Lucia makes an automatic assumption that her client would opt for surgery along with chemotherapy, since Lucia had described this as the most successful approach. Further, her client had spent a considerable amount of time during the initial interview talking about her children and how important it was for her to be involved with raising them and to see them graduated from high school. When Lucia spoke to her client to schedule the surgery and sign the operative forms, her client said that she must check with her husband since he may not want her to have surgery. She tells Lucia, "In my home, my husband makes all the decisions including what I should do about my cancer." Since Lucia firmly believes in a surgical approach for women with breast cancer, she talks to her client about the need to accept responsibility for her own health decisions.

Lucia does not meet this Standard since she believes that all women should share a common desire to protect their personal health. Lucia fails to recognize the importance of the Hispanic family's influence with respect to health decisions; the decision for surgery is no longer an individual choice. Lucia must learn to appreciate cultural diversity and the client/family's right to choose rather than to judge or fear that her client's husband will not make a decision that is appropriate for this family.

Standard of Practice 4.1.3

Holistic nurses explore with each person those strategies that can assist her/him, as desired, to understand the deeper meaning, purpose, inner strengths, and connections with self, others, nature, and God/Life Force/Absolute/Transcendent.

This Standard clearly emphasizes the importance in understanding the various dimensions of spirituality, and it suggests that nurses have a role in addressing the spiritual needs of clients. By acknowledging that individuals have health needs that encompass every dimension of their body-mind-spirit, nurses can assist their clients to be connected to their inner self, to others, to nature, and to God or higher power. Nurses who allow their spiritual being to surface and who become spiritual caregivers assist their clients to find meaning in life, illness, and suffering and they describe these experiences they share with clients as transformational events for both.[5] The nurse as a spiritual person and caregiver will assist clients in times of tragedy or great suffering.[6] He or she will be present in the moment, which means he or she will demonstrate a unique capacity for love, joy, caring, and compassion while assisting clients to have a hopeful perspective and offer hope when facing enormous challenges. It involves helping clients to grow and cope with life-threatening events and learning to find new ways of existing.[7]

Table 4–3 illustrates the nursing knowledge and skill required for a nurse to meet Standard 4.1.3.

Table 4–3 Interconnectedness in Holistic Nursing Practice

Standard of Practice 4.1.3	*Key Concepts*	*Requisite Knowledge*	*Requisite Skills*
Holistic nurses explore with each person those strategies that can assist her or him, as desired, to understand the deeper meaning, purpose, inner strengths, and connections with self, others, nature, and God/Life Force/Absolute/Transcendent.	Strategies to promote interconnectedness with self.	Theories of internal locus of control, self-perception; aligning with one's personal process of healing and unfolding.	Acceptance of self; acquire a realistic self-concept; recognize the unique gift of one's life; nurture one's growth to the fullest capacity.
	Strategies to promote interconnectedness with others.	Concepts of presence; conscious intention to appreciate the connection of the moment; giving of oneself freely.	Develop respect for each other and maintain healthy relationships; reinforce the strengths of the other person.
	Strategies to promote interconnectedness with nature.	Concepts related to the inherent healing rhythm of nature.	Engage in activities to be caretakers of the environment; know the natural environment is a gift from God.
	Strategies to promote interconnectedness with God/Life Force/Absolute/Transcendent.	Concepts related to communicating with a greater power; integrating an awareness of the meaning of life events, forgiveness of self or others.	Use of meditation, prayer, church attendance.

Nursing Activities

Nursing actions that demonstrate this Standard include: use of a spiritual assessment tool; use of strategies to nurture the spirit; defining goals of spiritual health; assisting clients to find meaning in life and illness or suffering; and ability to understand the meaning of prayer as an integral component of spirituality.

A spiritual assessment tool requires one to respond to a series of reflective questions that are aimed at assessing, evaluating, and increasing one's awareness of spirituality in self and others.[1] Used effectively, this tool can assist in the healing process. Using research as a means of discovery is also helpful in understanding the spiritual needs of others. For example, in speaking of the elements of spirituality, one study described how women view their spirituality as a source of inner strength. The findings showed how women spoke of things that mattered in life and how these things changed as the women journeyed over time. The most important revelation was the sense of connection with oneself, which included the essence of who one was, what and how one knows, and what one does and how one acts.[5] A second study, of the spirituality of patients recovering from acute myocardial infarction, had similar findings, clearly showing that spirituality was a life-giving force that came from within. "This life-giving force called spirituality was nurtured by receiving the presence of God, family, friends, and community." Furthermore, the findings in this study indicated that a person's perception of the meaning and purpose of spirituality that one held for his or her own life greatly influenced recovery from a major illness. Spirituality provided participants in this study with inner strength, comfort, peace, wellness, wholeness, and enhanced ability to cope.[6]

Using strategies to nurture the spirit involves taking time to experience the wonders of the world that surround us daily. (Some suggest that holistic nurses experience nature, living creatures, the earth that surrounds us, and Mother Earth.)[8] It means learning to relax, meditating or simply taking time to be centered. Walking outdoors, laughing, reading, and listening to music are also excellent ways to get in touch with one's own spirit. To nurture the spirit, one should also learn to form relationships with others, including extending oneself when needed to understand and accept even the most difficult relationships. To nurture the spirit, one should focus on the moment rather than live in the past or think only of the future.

To define effective goals for spiritual health, nurses must be mindful of what they do. It involves respecting others and being genuine; being compassionate and displaying human qualities of love, honesty, wisdom, and imagination. To define a goal for spirituality requires that nurses be fully present and able to understand the fear and pain experienced by their clients; they must learn to listen empathetically. Defining effective goals for spirituality also involves a willingness to pray with the clients if appropriate or to assist clients by helping them to interact with people who are a source of comfort, such as a minister, a priest, or a rabbi. Further, it means respecting a client's wish to use ritual, to attend prayer services, or to discover *God/Life Force/Absolute/Transcendent*'s call to wholeness.

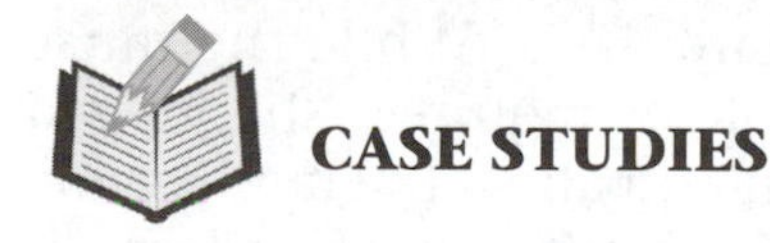

CASE STUDIES

1 Lisa, a hospice nurse, is visiting a 68-year-old client whose family has been told she probably has two weeks to two months to live. When Lisa enters the home, she finds Emmet, the client's husband, alone in the living room. He is very quiet and just seems to be staring without being focused or really looking at anything. He tells Lisa he does not want to be in the room with his wife because he is afraid of crying and he doesn't want his wife to see him upset. Emmet has only one daughter, and he feels he must also remain strong for her; he does not want his daughter to see him crying. Lisa offers support to Emmet by encouraging him to talk about his feelings of death. Lisa uses an open-ended question: "What do you see as your primary source of strength at the present time?" Lisa listens intently as Emmet expresses his fears and concerns about what is happening and how he will find strength. Emmet eventually reveals that it is not his crying that is stopping him from being at his wife's side; rather, he is angry at her for dying and he is ashamed of his feelings. He mentions how he and his wife did so much together. "We were best friends and inseparable; we did everything together whether the occasion was a vacation, a church fair, or a family reunion." Emmet talks of how close his wife and daughter are and how he fears his daughter will become depressed and lose interest in her job if something happens to his wife.

Lisa maintains a calm compassionate presence as Emmet tells his story. Lisa encourages Emmet to be at his wife's side; she helps Emmet to see that his wife would not be upset by his feelings but rather that she needed him to be there, to hold her hand, to pray with her, and that his presence might allow her to express her sadness at leaving his side.

Lisa meets Standard 4.1.3. A spiritual assessment revealed the client's relationship with her husband was built on closeness and sharing of experiences, which was a great source of comfort and strength to both of them in the past. Lisa facilitated a process to help Emmet articulate and find meaning in what was occurring at this moment. Lisa communicated an openness and a nonjudgmental attitude.

2 Janelle is preparing to go home from the hospital following the delivery of her stillborn baby. Janelle and her husband were both crying and Janelle tells her husband, "I have not slept well for the past two nights." In talking with the nurse, Janelle says, "How could this have happened to us? We went to all the prenatal classes and I was always in good health throughout my pregnancy. The baby was fine at my last checkup." The nurse listens intently and counsels the couple to find strength in each other. The nurse tells Janelle and her husband that this experience will make them stronger people; she suggests they talk to their minister because "God never gives anyone more than he or she can handle." In documenting her discharge note on Janelle's obstetrical record, the nurse writes the discharge diagnosis as "Ineffective family coping related to loss of a newborn as evidenced by crying and inability to sleep."

In this situation, the nurse does not meet Standard 4.1.3. While the nurse did listen intently and documented a discharge note as required, she judged the family's grieving inaccurately. Nurses must listen and allow the family time to grieve, and recognize that the grieving process is very personal and an essential step for future adaptation. Nurses must acknowledge a client's feelings without being judgmental or critical. Further, by responding to the client and her husband as she did, the nurse implied that "strength only comes with difficult situations such as the death of a baby." Additionally, nurses must avoid implying that because one is capable, he or she will be given more challenges. A more comforting response to this family's grieving would have been to say, "You are feeling sad and powerless and searching for a logical explanation for your loss." This response by the nurse would have supported a more realistic hope of finding meaning for the loss that Janelle and her husband suffered.

Standard of Practice 4.1.4

Holistic nurses recognize that holistic communication and awareness of individuals is a continuously evolving multi-level exchange that offers itself through dreams, images, symbols, sensations, meditations, and prayers.

This Standard underscores the value holistic nurses place on developing helping relationships using basic and advanced skills of communication. It is important to recognize that communication occurs within many dimensions, including extrasensory realms such as intuitive knowing and energetic vibrations.[2] Thus, when the helping relationship uses basic concepts of communication such as relaxation, imagery, or touch—or more advanced concepts based on biofeedback training or psychophysiology theory—communication with clients is improved.[1] It is also important to recognize that the use of methods such as relaxation and imagery teach an awareness of the direct link between body and emotions; it is a shift from body-mind-spirit split to body-mind integration.[9] This supports the use of interventions such as imagery before procedures to promote relaxation, which alters the physiological response and alleviates pain. Such techniques are also effective in relieving anxiety and increasing self-esteem.[10] Moreover, information gleaned from dreams, images, symbols, sensations, meditations, and prayers in general is therapeutic and leads to healthy dialogue and improved relationships.[1]

Table 4–4 illustrates the nursing knowledge and skill required for a nurse to meet Standard 4.1.4.

Table 4–4 The Multilevel Dimensions of Holistic Communication

Standard of Practice 4.1.4	*Key Concepts*	*Requisite Knowledge*	*Requisite Skills*
Holistic nurses recognize that holistic communication and awareness of individuals is a continuously evolving multi-level exchange that offers itself through dreams, images, symbols, sensations, meditations, and prayers.	The multi-level dimensions of holistic communication.	Knowledge of physiologic responses to stress; knowledge of basic and advanced techniques of relaxation.	Ability to integrate healing/caring strategies and healing reflections for self and others; ability to remain in the present moment, to use advanced communication skills.
	Finding meaning in symbols, dreams, images, sensations, meditation, and prayer.	Concepts of communication supporting intuitive knowing, searching for meaning, awareness.	Interventions using dreams, images, symbols, sensations, meditation, and prayer.

Nursing Activities

Nursing actions that demonstrate this Standard include: interventions that empower self and others to recognize the importance of caring for the body-mind-spirit by using relaxation techniques; using strategies to facilitate and interpret the imagery process; and/or using advanced skills in psychophysiology of body-mind healing.

Practical strategies for immediate relaxation include interventions that are aimed at "letting go" of the effects of unwanted stress. Holistic nurses learn to assess and give meaning to the communication between mind and body as expressed in thoughts, attitudes, feelings, and emotions. For example, when one becomes aggravated or angry, with subsequent elevation in blood pressure, using the more basic techniques such as breathing exercises, slowing the rate of speech, releasing muscle tension, or practicing nondefensive responses are all useful ways to relieve anxiety. Music therapy is often used to calm inner thoughts and feelings of stress. Similarly, a very effective way of restoring energy and at the same time getting to know who you are is to meditate. Nurses need to encourage their clients to take the time for solitude or spiritual contemplation.[7]

Imagery or visualization is a process of mentally picturing an event that you wish to have occur in the present or future. It is an equally important process to improve communication skills; it can be used alone or in combination with other relaxation techniques. With imagery, nurses learn to produce positive healing results that, when implemented effectively for self or others, have been shown to decrease stress and increase feelings of confidence and competence.[11,12] Imagery allows inner silence, inward focusing, and a sense of mastery along with the ability to increase psychophysiologic healing.

Many different types of imagery have been identified, and their success is based on clearly defining the outcome prior to the intervention.[1] For example, end state imagery is the rehearsal of being in a final, healed state. (The client who is recovering from a myocardial infarction sees himself well with a healthy heart, exercising regularly and returning to work.) Interactive guided imagery goes to an even deeper level of eliciting and using a person's own images, both positive and negative. (A client's menstrual cycle is lengthened and premenstrual distress is reduced.)[11] Equally important is the use of techniques such as reframing for empowering imagery scripts. (A client states she has always had poor circulation in her legs, with aching arthritic-like cramps since she was a young girl. All medical testing has shown there is no underlying physical reason for the client to suffer leg pain, yet it seems to occur whenever she is under undue stress. With reframing, the client is instructed to say, "My leg veins are not constricted, my legs are healthy and I can feel the warmth of the blood flow freely through my veins.") It is important to help the client to change a long-held belief by reassociating or reorganizing his or her experience of pain in a manner that establishes a healthier state.[1]

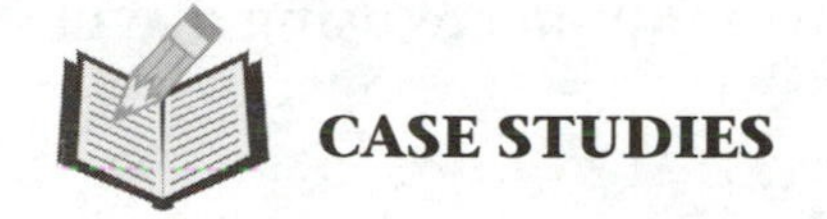

CASE STUDIES

1 As a nurse manager, you are starting a new task for the day, writing a summary report for your department that is due by the end of the day. Before you begin, a letter written by a colleague is brought to your attention—it is an inflammatory response to activities that occurred during a recent team meeting. You immediately feel angry and you feel your muscles tense in a fight-flight response. However, as a holistic nurse you have come to value the ability to practice relaxation techniques in the face of unexpected stressful events. You begin an on-the-spot relaxation technique, viewing yourself reclining in a hot bath, the jets of the whirlpool spraying soothing water that relaxes your muscles. The steam from the hot water clouds your glasses and you close your eyes as you let each muscle from your head and neck to your toes relax. You feel your mind release the tension; you have calm and inner self-confidence, you are strengthened and energized. When you open your eyes, you realize that your energies need to be free to write your report, which is your priority action. You have successfully met Standard 4.1.4.

2 Loretta is a 29-year-old recently diagnosed with chronic systemic lupus. Her friends have helped her learn about the illness from reading materials they found on the Internet or at the local bookstore. Loretta reads fervently but finds she is quickly overwhelmed by all the complications she is likely to experience. Soon, Loretta begins to exhibit increasing physical symptoms along with some signs of possible clinical depression. She searches for help at the clinic where she receives care but finds her doctors are unsympathetic. She is placed on medication and told to resume her daily routine and enjoy her family. Unsatisfied with this care, Loretta asks her friends to help her find a nurse healer familiar with relaxation and imagery techniques. Loretta visits this nurse healer, who teaches her about the psychobiology of mind-body healing. She is guided through an incredible journey in her own immune system where she awakens the healing forces that will clear her body of invading blood cells. Loretta envisions a light shining into her own DNA; this light guides the unwanted *B* cells from her body.

By assisting clients using guided imagery techniques, the nurse healer helps clients find inner resources to control pain, enhance the immune function, and to remove or modify barriers that prevent them from being successful in using imagery. The nurse healer meets Standard 4.1.4. She assesses Loretta to be a good candidate because of her strong imagination. Further, she assists Loretta to visualize how she wants to see her body recover and helps her to take action to make it happen. The nurse assists Loretta in the healing process not only by helping her gain new knowledge about her own psychophysiological responses but also by showing her how to know herself in a new way. Loretta and her nurse learned to communicate using a symbolic language.[1]

Standard of Practice 4.1.5

Holistic nurses respect the person's health trajectory, which may be incongruent with conventional wisdom.

This Standard dictates that nurses understand the health belief systems of self and others and respect alternate ways of knowing and choosing. Everyone and every body is unique; because of that, various experiences in one's healing journey, in combination with cultural factors and learned behaviors, greatly impact one's beliefs about health-wellness-disease-illness. Consequently, one develops patterns and behaviors that impact the whole human health experience, from the perspective of how one perceives well-being to the meaning and significance ascribed to an experience of illness. This Standard implies that holistic nurses not only recognize the important distinctions between disease and individual illness experience but have the responsibility to help their clients understand the distinctions as well. Further, this Standard implies that nurses recognize that determining the health status of the client within the context of that client's values is essential in providing a framework for planning, implementing, and evaluating outcomes of care.

Table 4–5 illustrates the nursing knowledge and skill required for a nurse to meet Standard 4.1.5.

Table 4–5 Health Choices in Holistic Practice

Standard of Practice 4.1.5	*Key Concepts*	*Requisite Knowledge*	*Requisite Skills*
Holistic nurses respect the person's health trajectory, which may be incongruent with conventional wisdom.	Health trajectory.	Concepts of health-wellness and disease-illness.	Engage in holistic practice within the context of a person's cultural background, health beliefs, and values.
	Self-determination.	Knowledge of empowerment; concepts related to independent decision making and self-responsibility.	Strategies to support client autonomy.
	Conventional wisdom; alternate ways of knowing and choosing.	Customary, traditional practices of Western medicine; alternative therapies.	Methods of care in agreement with allopathic models.

Nursing Activities

Nursing actions that demonstrate this Standard include respect for the use of the customary, traditional practices of Western medicine and mind-oriented therapies of holistic care, as the client chooses.

The key to competent holistic care is demonstrated when nurses respect the client's decision about his or her own health. For many individuals, modern medicine has been successful in fighting some illnesses even though many diseases are yet to be conquered. Based on the perceived benefits of modern medicine, most clients still choose a conventional approach to care. This means their medical therapy may surround the use of state-of-the-art technology in determining diagnoses, prescription medications, specialized treatments and/or surgery along with expensive hospital stays when illness presents complex health problems. Yet even with these advanced approaches, access is not available to all. Further, many Americans do not receive good or even adequate health care supervision. This results in many individuals becoming dissatisfied and feeling modern medicine does little to prevent illness or deal with lifestyle problems such as stress, addiction, and even weight problems associated with the fast-paced life of contemporary America. As a consequence, clients are becoming more receptive to alternative or nontraditional health care approaches. They actively seek out practitioners who specialize in therapies such as bodywork, herbal medicine, or imagery.

Throughout the process of determining one's course of care, holistic nurses ensure that attention is paid to the caring aspect and not merely a focus on curing and cost in providing care. Further, holistic nurses respect and use all possible resources to assist clients to achieve optimum levels of well-being. This often requires that interventions used are complementary, such as the use of alternative modalities alone or in combinations with conventional methods of care. Both the allopathic and alternative approaches to care emphasize wellness with the client as active participant in the healing process and in maintaining a harmonious balance of body, mind, and spirit.

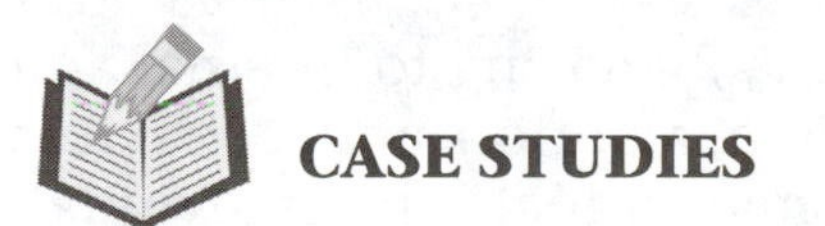

CASE STUDIES

1 Shirley was admitted to the medical center with a diagnosis of melanoma. Her condition was determined to be critical since the cancer had metastasized to her kidneys, liver, and lungs. The physicians wanted to treat the cancer aggressively because Shirley was still very young and a very active member of a prominent family in town. They explained that with treatment she could live for six to eight months, but without it her chances of being alive in three months were very poor. Shirley's choice was to forgo the chemotherapy since she believed it would alter the quality of time she had remaining on this earth. Her goal was to be free of the physical discomforts that the treatments would cause. Shirley shared with her nurse that she wanted to be kept comfortable but alert enough to communicate with her family. She asked for certain foods and drinks. The nurse frequently brought Shirley herbal drinks and taught her a self-care technique using meditation.

The nurse meets Standard 4.1.5 because she respects and supports Shirley's choice for alternative therapy. In addition, the nurse helps Shirley to achieve a spiritual calm and heightened awareness after each meditation session.

2 Billy is a 48-year-old bus driver recently diagnosed with high blood pressure. The occupational health nurse sees him on a weekly basis because of his high blood pressure and for physical therapy to his left arm, which was injured from the immobilization of the arm following a clavicle fracture. The health assessment that the nurse completed reveals Billy smokes cigars daily and his wife smokes close to one pack of cigarettes per day. Because his job is stressful, he is overweight and he gets very little exercise. The nurse recommends that he change his health-related behaviors now. However, Billy and his wife face many other life stresses because of their autistic son and other difficulties with their two daughters. Billy, who has smoked since he was 13 years of age, chooses not to add additional stress to his life by attempting to change his smoking behaviors. The nurse insists that Billy change his ways before it is too late and he suffers a stroke. She counsels him weekly about his lifestyle and cautions that he also needs to convince his wife to change, since secondhand smoke is as dangerous.

The nurse does not meet this Standard since she fails to accept that Billy is entitled to make his own lifestyle choices even when they are incongruent with recommended health behaviors.

4.2 Therapeutic Environment

■■ Holistic nurses recognize that each person's environment includes everything that surrounds the individual, both the external and internal (physical, mental, emotional, social, and spiritual) as well as patterns not yet understood. ■■

The concept of environment is multidimensional, referring to internal and external factors that influence an individual's perception and behaviors throughout life. It includes everything that may impact an individual, whether it is from a physical, social, psychological, cultural, or spiritual dimension. Nurses are often reminded how they must understand the world that surrounds their clients, how they must convey a caring and compassionate attitude in order to create a therapeutic environment. Think of the lonely unresponsive person who delights in the presence of an animal. In like manner, the condition of an extremely ill person in the intensive care unit stabilizes once a caring encounter is established to help lessen external stimuli and assist him or her to maintain a sense of self in a bewildering situation. Nurses who show concern for the client as a person and who have a sensitive awareness of the client's needs or what he or she is experiencing in his or her personal environment create a therapeutic relationship, a therapeutic environment.

When reflecting on the concept of environment and the natural world, the direct relationship between human health and environmental quality cannot be underscored. For example, when nurses consider their clients and the environment, they must give thought to global issues such as population growth, limited resources, and climate changes contributing to increased exposure to illnesses. Furthermore, halting the spread of infectious disease, dealing with issues of poor nutrition, eliminating poverty, or attempting to preserve environmental resources are all important to promoting a healthy environment. When considering how to resolve the issues related to environment from the perspective of the world that surrounds people, holistic nurses are encouraged to focus on self-responsible behavior by not contributing to potential health problems of others (smoking in public areas, washing with solvents). In addition holistic nurses must act accountably by participating in socially responsible activities such as recycling or speaking out to control hazardous waste sites. It is important to always remember that human beings and their world cannot be separated.

In like manner, quality of life issues related to personal protection cannot be overemphasized. Accepting responsibility to protect one's surroundings has prompted an even greater awareness, among holistic nurses, as to how one's external environment impacts one's internal responses whether this is a physical, immune system response or a psychological response to increased levels of stress. In addition, research findings have shown that others do affect the surroundings of many, for example, as seen with secondhand cigarette smoke or stale air. Likewise, inanimate things affect one's well-being, such as environmental noises from household appliances or inadequate lighting. Irradiation of food products is an equally controversial topic rated as high as worker's safety issues that resulted in national attention with the passage of legislation to protect employees from hazardous chemicals or the effects of asbestos or latex products. Whether as citizens, employees, or entrepreneurs, nurses are in a strategic position to influence public policy related to environmental problems that are systemic problems, interconnected and interdependent.[13]

Standard of Practice 4.2.1

Holistic nurses promote environments conducive to experiencing healing, wholeness, and harmony, and care for the person in as healthy an environment as possible.

This Standard emphasizes the nurses' responsibility to be aware that a person cannot be fully understood without an analysis of the environment that supports or compromises his or her existence. This analysis must go well beyond simply viewing the tangible physical setting or the internal and external factors surrounding an individual or his or her immediate family. It mandates that psychosocial environmental factors—such as perception of one's well-being, family support, social norms, culture, and religion—be considered as well, since they also play a major role in one's ability to heal and to have inner harmony and peace of mind.

Table 4–6 illustrates the nursing knowledge and skill required for a nurse to meet Standard 4.2.1.

Table 4–6 Health Environments for Healing

Standard of Practice 4.2.1	*Key Concepts*	*Requisite Knowledge*	*Requisite Skills*
Holistic nurses promote environments conducive to experiencing healing, wholeness, and harmony, and care for the person in as healthy an environment as possible.	Healthy environments.	Concepts related to building a healthy environment, including one's personal and planetary home.	Expand awareness of psychosocial environmental elements, environmental hazards; role model–responsible behavior; support socially responsible environmental groups.
	Promoting environments conducive to healing, wholeness, and harmony.	Concepts related to life-sustaining practices and healing interventions.	Use of respectful, healing treatments and appropriate caring methods such as intuitive knowing and empathy, professional competence, supporting the patient's integrity, prayer, healing services, or reminiscence.

Nursing Activities

Nursing actions that demonstrate this Standard include using the nursing process with environment as the client to prevent problems before they occur. Many people are unaware of the influences existing within an environmental setting. Lately, people have focused on the hazards associated with secondhand smoke, but very little attention is directed at diminishing or eliminating a myriad of bad habits that can pose a health risk in later life. Since nurses provide care in and across all environments, they focus not only on the individual's level of health care but also manage, monitor, and manipulate the surrounding environment to foster health. For example, in thinking of the child's world, what he or she sees at home can reduce the effectiveness of the best health education program implemented in school. That is, if the child is exposed to drugs or sees adverse sexual behavior in the home, the child is likely to develop these habits as well. Similarly, when a child is brought up in a home where physical exercise, good nutrition, or healthy dental care is not practiced, the child will be at risk for obesity and other health-related illness in adulthood.

An equally important responsibility for holistic nurses is to increase awareness of the meaning of environmental space. Nurses are keenly aware of the need to provide privacy when interviewing a client about a recent rape or when performing invasive procedures. Likewise, nurses will often assess the need for proper lighting, ventilation, or tolerable noise levels. Yet nurses often fail to seek the meaning of environment in relation to the client's desire for sacred space—that is, the quiet space for personal prayer or meditation. Identifying client outcomes adequately creates a psychological environment that supports healing and fosters safe interpersonal relationships.

CASE STUDIES

1 Benjamin, an 84-year-old minister, is recovering from major surgery and has recently been told that he will have to enter a nursing home, probably for the remainder of his life since he has no family able to care for him at home. Benjamin knew he would eventually be unable to care for himself at home, but he had prayed his life would take a different turn so that this type of living arrangement could be avoided.

The nurse supervisor is aware of Benjamin's stress related to being a nursing home resident. Further, she knows that he has requested a sacred space to meditate and pray. Because the nurse wants to facilitate a comfortable transition for Benjamin, she takes extra precautions to prepare Benjamin's room and ensure it is free of all noxious stimuli that might be upsetting to him. She checks to be sure the television is turned off and the window opened slightly to allow fresh air to circulate. The room has been freshly painted with soft colors, and all bed linens and curtains match to create a pleasant environmental space. The nurse meets Standard 4.2.1.

2 Gloria is a nurse manager for a firm who will be building a new assisted living facility in town. Gloria has been asked to participate on a planning committee. Her major responsibility is to recommend an ideal environment for a resident's living quarters. Thus her plan is to convey the importance of environmental quality, to stress the healing benefits of sound, color, light, fresh air, warmth, and cleanliness. For example, her plan is to talk of nature, meaning all rooms need a window; personal space, meaning all rooms should be private rooms; social support, meaning there must be a place for visitors' comfort; color, meaning the hues must be soothing; sounds, meaning to provide a peaceful environment with control of music, TV, and call bells—which is particularly important when one's living arrangements are shared by many others. Conversely, stimulation is a critical element in caring for the elderly; thus there must be space to provide for diversion and activity to prevent loneliness and depression.

The nurse meets Standard 4.2.1 because she is aware and sensitive to the interconnections of environment and the quality of human living.

Standard of Practice 4.2.2

Holistic nurses work toward creating organizations that value sacred space and environments that enhance healing.

The Standard relates to organizations that not only value sacred space, a quiet place to explore life's meaning, but organizations whose members share similar values, have a common vision, and work toward the common goal of healing themselves in order to heal the ailing and failing health care system. It is not uncommon to hear individuals who share similar beliefs say that they and their colleagues are "like minded." Members of the American Holistic Nurses' Association (AHNA) share this oneness; they have similar philosophical beliefs and are guided by standards of professional practice. Members of AHNA support caring experiences for all that can be transformational events bringing about healing and growth toward wholeness, even in the midst of devastating crisis or death. An example of a shared value has been clearly conceptualized in clinical practice through the work of holistic practitioners who view nurses as the environment for the client leading to a healing experience. This theory puts forth the view that when nurses expand their own consciousness, they become the healing environment for the client. In becoming a sacred space, nurses also are healed.[14]

Table 4–7 illustrates the nursing knowledge and skill required for a nurse to meet Standard 4.2.2.

Table 4–7 Sacred Space and Healing Environments

Standard of Practice 4.2.2	*Key Concepts*	*Requisite Knowledge*	*Requisite Skills*
Holistic nurses work toward creating organizations that value sacred space and environments that enhance healing.	Holistic organizations.	Organizational philosophy; membership development, common purpose and goals for creating wellness.	Resources and leadership abilities to connect and guide professional groups in similar directions.
	Sacred space.	Practices associated with creating healing environments—external and relationship focused.	Ability to embrace healing environments.
	Environments that enhance healing.	Concepts related to personal and community space environments.	Engage in activities to provide safety education; global safety, handling toxic substances, and issues within the workplace.

Nursing Activities

Nursing actions that demonstrate this Standard include a willingness to join professional associations, engaging in personal and professional development activities, or maintaining an affiliation with specialty groups who share similar goals for care.

Holism in nursing is the foundational concept to uphold for members of AHNA who view their role as therapeutic partners with the client. The major responsibility for holistic nurses is to promote health, facilitate healing, and alleviate suffering. An example of how holistic nurses would interpret this goal can be heard in their view of pain and suffering. Pain and suffering are not seen as bad and health as good; rather, holistic nurses see both as natural events and necessary components of lifelong growth and learning and movement toward self-awareness and wellness.[14]

Many nurses are also committed to taking advantage of educational opportunities to enhance one's knowledge and practice of holistic nursing. For example, many seek certification through the American Holistic Nurses Certification Corporation (AHNCC) as a way of demonstrating excellence in practice. For holistic nurses, the educational opportunities allow one to earn continuing education credit in a multitude of ways by attending national, local, or regional conferences or seminars or through independent study. Similarly, many nurses take advantage of certificate programs such as the Certificate Program in Holistic Nursing. Many choose to be certified in certain healing modalities; thus they might seek certification from Healing Touch Programs, Aromatherapy for Health Professionals, Nurse Certificate Program in Imagery, or The National Nurses' Certificate Program in AMMA Therapy. Many nurses are licensed RN Massage Therapists, while others gain additional education and practice in specialty fields such as Biofeedback, Herbal Medicine, Hypnotherapy, Reflexology, and Vitamin and Mineral Therapy.

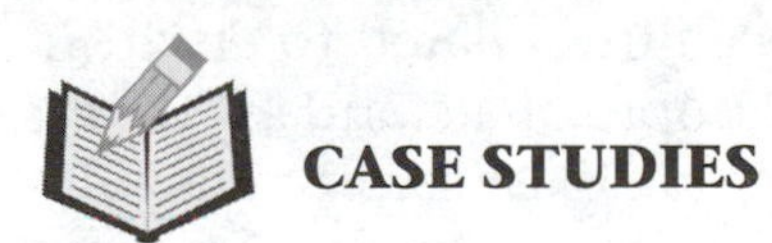

CASE STUDIES

1 Bonnie, a member of AHNA, is in private practice in Nashville. She volunteers as a Regional Coordinator for AHNA in Tennessee, helping spread the word about holistic nursing. Bonnie is also a member of the Tennessee Nurses Association. In her practice, Bonnie provides holistic nursing care in the form of energetic healing and wellness counseling and education. She recently published an article, "Holistic Nursing: A Breed of Its Own," in the *Tennessee Nurse.*[15] Bonnie exemplifies the qualities desired of holistic nurses, and she meets Standard 4.2.2 through her nursing practice, professional involvement, and publications. She demonstrates the leadership abilities to connect and guide professional groups in similar directions while at the same time assists her peers by helping them to understand what holistic nursing is and how it differs from non-holistic nursing.

2 Melissa is a nurse who is dedicated to her clients. Her ability to carry out her role is intertwined with her self-concept; thus she is extremely cautious to focus on this aspect of care in working with clients. She assesses the meaning of role. For example, she recently worked with a young athlete who was injured in a motorcycle accident and who is now a quadriplegic. Her goal is to assist this client to gain a new sense of role. Her assessment focuses on his developmental stage, available resources, and social networks. In addition, she makes sure to identify the client's understanding of the effect of this injury on his abilities to meet his self-care needs and the possible ways his injuries may impact his relationships with others.

When discussing her goals and plan of care for her client with the other nurses on her unit, Melissa is complimented on being a client advocate and competent in providing quality care. One of her colleagues asks Melissa if she would share her skills with others by presenting an inservice for nurses from the local district of the state nurses' association. Melissa declines the invitation, saying she has difficulty speaking in public. When asked if she belonged to any professional associations, she said she cannot afford the dues money and needed to be with her children at night as opposed to being out with friends.

In this instance, Melissa is a qualified clinical nurse but she does not meet Standard 4.2.2. Melissa is reluctant to participate or share her knowledge with members of a professional organization who come together in common purpose and whose goals are to promote the advancement of the profession of nursing through a sharing of knowledge and expertise.

Standard of Practice 4.2.3

Holistic nurses integrate holistic principles, standards, policies, and procedures in relation to environmental safety and emergency preparedness.

The Standard underscores the holistic nurse's responsibility to base his or her practice on holistic principles, standards of care, and Standards of Practice. By way of illustration, integrating policies and procedures related to environmental safety and emergency preparedness is an example of a standard that is foundational to one's holistic practice. Standards of care exist to provide guidance to nurses in practice and to define appropriate levels of quality of client care. Holistic nurses are expected to know and follow these Standards of Practice. The nurse's performance related to environmental safety and emergency preparedness assists the nurse to assess the severity of the situation (major disaster, worker's safety, an attempted suicide) and the client's danger potential. During the intervention phase, the nurse acts as an advocate, resource, partner, and guide to the client, assisting him or her to mobilize personal strengths and to use support persons and resources effectively. The emergency protocols, policies, and procedures of the setting guide the nurse's actions and assist the nurse to give focused, attentive, and intensive care during the "crisis" situation.

Table 4–8 illustrates the nursing knowledge and skill required for a nurse to meet Standard 4.2.3.

Table 4–8 Environmental Safety and Emergency Preparedness

Standard of Practice 4.2.3	*Key Concepts*	*Requisite Knowledge*	*Requisite Skills*
Holistic nurses integrate holistic principles, standards, policies, and procedures in relation to environmental safety and emergency preparedness.	Holistic principles, standards, policies, and procedures.	Concepts related to the art and science of nursing, intuitive and analytical skills, and interconnectedness of body, mind, and spirit.	Use of healing caring interventions in practice based on holistic Standards of Care and the holistic Standards of Practice.
	Environmental safety.	Theory related to the influence of surroundings on the health and welfare of an individual or groups of people.	Engage in activities to assess the impact of one's problem on environmental safety; implement safety education programs.
	Emergency preparedness.	Theory and practice related to anticipating the potential effect of environmental hazards or life-threatening factors associated with emergencies such as earthquakes, tornadoes, hurricanes.	Policy and procedure related to environmental safety and elimination of harmful elements; emergency plans to respond in times of major disasters.

Nursing Activities

Nursing actions that demonstrate this Standard include increasing awareness of environmental space and environmental hazards, and committing to use environmental interventions to improve quality care and reduce hazards.

Everything that surrounds an individual or group of people impacts them in some way; whether this brings a positive or negative response depends on the causative factor. For example, soothing music in the environment can be relaxing. Waiting on the phone to connect to a "live person" is often more acceptable when music is played in the background. However, when something in the environment is an actual or potential threat, it is hazardous to one's well-being—for example, environmental toxins or food allergens can render one ill. Nurses play an important role in assisting clients with an environmental illness by helping them find new ways to adjust. In one scenario, a client may need to be taught how to keep a food diary if illness seems to erupt after ingestion of certain foods. Whether the allergy is from the food product or a possible toxin used during the growing period will have to be determined. Showing the client how to track symptoms and record foods eaten during a "trial and error period" can be very beneficial in helping the client determine the cause of the symptoms and contribute to the related medical diagnosis.

Stress in the environment is also known to impact one's internal environment. Many individuals are known to suffer clinical depression, particularly in the winter months when short days contribute to loneliness and seclusion. Because the response to a particular environmental stress varies greatly, identifying the cause of the symptom or the pattern of behavior is critical. Nurses have a responsibility to evaluate a person's home environment, work situation, and family relationships to detect the possible influences each has in contributing to his or her illness. Moreover, nurses have a responsibility to educate the person and his or her significant family members as to the possible contributing factors that impinge on their health and lead to illness.

Sometimes the environmental hazard is not easily controlled. For example, infectious diseases can easily spread and infect hundreds of people in one small community. Toxic waste alters the natural world that everyone shares. The nurse's responsibility in such situations surrounds the need to conduct an exposure survey. In some instances, the responsibility would probably lie in what the nurse does as a consumer and the individual choices he or she makes. Refusing to buy items that are served in styrofoam packages is an example. Still, in other situations, the nurse may be taking a proactive stance in lobbying for legislation to change the way we conduct business—for example, requiring labeling of food products that have been genetically altered.

CASE STUDIES

1 Joyce, a school nurse, is concerned about the smoking that goes on in the teacher's lounge. There is also a second room that is quite smoked-filled; this is the room where students congregate for school-related meetings. Concerned about the smokers' health and the health of the innocent students who are exposed to secondhand smoke, Joyce decides to seek change in the school policy. She drafts a revised policy for a smoke-free environment and brings the policy to the school board. Needless to say, Joyce is outraged when the policy was defeated. Not wishing to abandon her desire to see change, Joyce talks to her principal, also a nonsmoker, to see what she should have done differently. Talks with the principal revealed that the chairman of the school board has a sister who is a teacher at the school, a teacher who smokes close to one pack of cigarettes per day.

Joyce changes her strategy and seeks the support of other teachers and students who are nonsmokers. They hold focus groups and discuss the pros and cons of designated smoke areas versus a smoke-free environment. Joyce also holds focus groups with some of the parent groups. The first meetings were rather caustic, as the smokers showed up in force at all of these small focus groups to protest any change.

Determined to make an impact, Joyce drafted a new policy; however, this time she offered to start smoking-cessation classes. Further, she invited many of the parents to attend the board meeting with her. She also had a 50-year-old man who is oxygen dependent and suffering from Chronic Obstructive Pulmonary Disease (COPD) with her. The school board members were silent during this presentation, yet focused on the man with COPD. Many wondered whether that would be them in future years or, for that matter, if this was what would happen to their children. The second policy passed unanimously and the schools in Joyce's district are all smoke-free buildings. Joyce meets Standard 4.2.3.

2 Bettie, a home health nurse, is documenting her nursing interventions following a visit to a young mother of two children, including one four-year-old child who has multiple sclerosis. During her visit, Bettie noticed that Brian, the 11-month-old child, was kept in the playpen throughout the visit. In conversation, Bettie learned that Brian is beginning to walk and climb. His mother fears he will injure himself in a fall or get into household products under the sink, so for his safety, she keeps him in the playpen all day. The young mother reported that she is extremely busy with her disabled child, and Brian seems to have adjusted to this confinement since he is able to amuse himself. The mother reports Brian cries only when he is wet or hungry.

Bettie's documentation focuses only on the interventions she had with the child who has multiple sclerosis. She did not pursue any further discussion with the mother relative to the 11-month-old, nor did she recommend further follow-up care for young Brian.

In this case study, Bettie does not meet Standard 4.2.3. Maintaining safety in the environment is very important, but there must be a balance between safety precautions and quality of life. Brian's growth and development needs require that he not be restricted from movement. A priority assessment would have been to determine if this young mother was spending an excessive amount of time with the disabled child to the exclusion of meeting the needs of the 11-month-old. Additionally, inquiring whether there were others such as family, friends, or neighbors who could assist in the care of the disabled child would have allowed respite for the mother. Referrals to community agencies for daycare supervision could have been investigated. An additional intervention could have been to assist this young mother in recognizing how to balance priorities for both children. Discussing overall care needs of an 11-month-old with respect to strengthening leg muscles or foot development or supporting the development of curiosity could have been part of Bettie's plan of care even if many of the interventions were suggested for follow-up visits. Education plans could have focused on how to provide a safe environment for toddlers.

Standard of Practice 4.2.4

Holistic nurses recognize that the well-being of the ecosystem of the planet is a prior determining condition for the well-being of the human.

This Standard relates to health and the natural world; it highlights the nurse's responsibility to consider the health of the ecosystem in relation to the need for health, safety, inner harmony, and peace for all persons. Many profound changes have impacted the world we live in. To illustrate, there are many more people in this world, people are living longer, people move into large cities, people are more culturally diverse, and they travel to and from faraway countries. Further, there are fewer natural resources available. Water is fast becoming a scarce commodity, and in many areas, water sources are contaminated and land is scarce. Based on this information, holistic nurses recognize their responsibility to detect possible environmental influences on their clients' illnesses, knowing that a wide range of effects caused by environmental toxins, as one example, can contribute to complex disease states.

Significant changes in the climate are also contributing to a global warming. This adds to major health-related illnesses, with more outbreaks of infectious disease, and mass destruction of land and lives from earthquakes, hurricanes, tornadoes, floods, fire, and deforestation. Nurses have a major responsibility to be proactive in educating the public with respect to the dangers inherent in the world around them. The importance of public health education, ensuring vaccinations to those in need, cannot be overstated. Equally important is the need to be actively involved in local stewardship of the land around one's community. Holistic nurses can protect the environment by role modeling and participating in a recycling program. This is a simple yet effective way to demonstrate concerned citizenship.

Table 4–9 illustrates the nursing knowledge and skill required for a nurse to meet Standard 4.2.4.

Table 4–9 Healthy Ecosystems for Well-Being

Standard of Practice 4.2.4	*Key Concepts*	*Requisite Knowledge*	*Requisite Skills*
Holistic nurses recognize that the well-being of the ecosystem of the planet is a prior determining condition for the well-being of the human.	Healthy ecosystem.	Awareness and knowledge of environmental factors that impact the natural world.	Use of practical ways to cope with hazards in the environment.
	Conditions to promote well-	Theories and research about direct links between	Engage in activities to promote safety in the workplace;

continues

Table 4–9 continued

Standard of Practice 4.2.4	*Key Concepts*	*Requisite Knowledge*	*Requisite Skills*
	being in humankind.	environmental hazards and human response patterns.	promote consciousness raising related to safe food, safe water, Maternal-Child Health services; safety in the schools.

Nursing Activities

Nursing actions that demonstrate this Standard include environmental assessment-exposure survey, and use of the nursing process with environment as client, with person as client.

Nurses can engage in activities to protect the ecosystem of the planet by assessing and evaluating the environment and focusing on ecological problems, particularly those identified by the two federal agencies, the Environmental Protection Agency (EPA) and Occupational Safety and Health Administration (OSHA). The problems identified by the EPA include but are not limited to changes in the global climate, indoor as well as outside air pollutants, and toxic air such as carbon monoxide or the effects of smog. Other problems focus on radon gas, ozone depletion, use of pesticides, and occupational exposure to chemicals.[13] OSHA monitors the environment relative to workplace health hazards. The "Right to Know" Act protects workers and requires employers to notify individuals of possible hazards. Further, this law requires the employer to provide education regarding safe use of toxic substances along with maintaining health records on all individuals who are routinely exposed.[1]

Completing an environmental survey is often difficult simply because there are so many intervening variables that impact the client's health. However, even the smallest amount of information can help to detect those substances or lifestyle factors that are capable of bringing on untoward reactions in people. Moreover, the information gained from environmental surveys is helpful in planning education programs that can assist clients to learn how to eliminate or modify those factors that contribute to illness or chronic disease. To illustrate: When environment is viewed as client, the perspective of interconnections between human and environment is understood. Nurses caring for clients with leukemia are acting responsibly when they also become actively involved in community issues pertaining to toxic dumpsites. The community and broader environment become the client. While nurses attempt to bring about change within the community, they share their knowledge of the impact of these community problems on the health and well-being of their clients. Counseling clients with leukemia may include information on location of toxic waste sites or even referrals to help clients relocate if they happen to live in close proximity to a dumpsite. Beyond completing surveys, nurses need to conduct research relative to environmental problems to determine the effect they have on one's health.

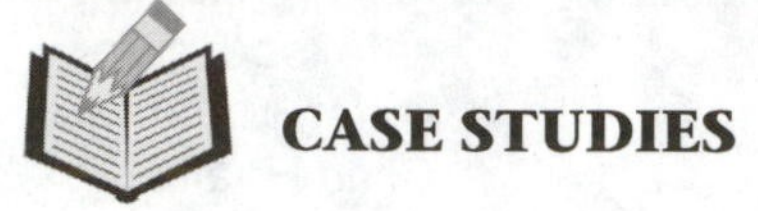

CASE STUDIES

1 Noise pollution has been identified by many as contributing to hearing problems, irritability, and anxiety. Some studies have even shown that productivity at work is diminished if the noise reaches hazardous levels. Knowing this, Sherry, a nursing supervisor at a local nursing home, has set about to bring change on the unit. Sherry suspects that the nurses on the unit are contributing to resident health problems and they are not even aware of it. The problem that Sherry has identified relates to those residents who are chairbound, easily agitated, fidgety, and unable to interact with other residents in recreational activities. These residents do not feed themselves and they require complete care to meet their personal hygiene needs. Because close supervision is required, these residents are usually brought to the nurses' station and sit for long periods of time in their wheelchairs. The nurses' station is usually a very active environment and, to complicate matters, nurses put a radio or TV on to keep the residents stimulated. Before long, three different shifts of nurses have been on duty and it can be recorded that the resident has spent most of his/her waking hours, and possibly some nighttime hours, at the nurses' station. The danger posed by noise pollution is a function of the volume of sound heard over a period of time.[1] Volume of sound, in this instance, is not only from the radio or TV, but it also comes from the constant noise associated with talking by the workers, the buzzing sound of the call bells, and the ring of the telephone.

Sherry conducts a research study, looking at outcomes of care for those residents who are cared for in quieter environments compared to those behaviors and patterned responses of the residents who sit at the nurses' station for long periods of time. The findings support Sherry's theory. Residents who are cared for in quieter environments have a more restful sleep pattern, require less medication for restlessness, eat regular meals with less assistance, and are more willing to interact at recreational activities. Sherry meets Standard 4.2.4.

2 Kyle is a 25-year-old unemployed laborer. He has just been called to do a job that involves removal of asbestos from an old building that will be converted into apartments for low-income couples. Kyle is a hard worker but his educational background has been disadvantaged so his reading skills and level of understanding are limited. Consequently, Kyle has heard very little about the dangers of working with asbestos. The company has provided an orientation but they do little to verify that Kyle understands the dangers he could face

from simply breathing in the particles from the asbestos if he removes his mask. A second potentially hazardous factor is that Kyle has been diagnosed with Crohn's disease and has frequent bouts with diarrhea. Kyle is seen at the clinic for a pre-employment physical and he tells the nurse about his new job. Nurse Amy congratulates Kyle and wishes him well, saying he must feel good now that he will have a regular income.

Nurse Amy does not meet Standard 4.2.4. First, she fails to ask any questions to determine how much Kyle knows of the dangers associated with asbestos. Second, Amy does not warn him about picking up heavy objects; an activity that, when done frequently, usually contributes to aggravate symptoms related to Crohn's disease. Working with asbestos removal frequently involves lifting heavy objects. Third, Amy does not have information about safety education programs at the company, nor does she suggest that Kyle attempt to find out which education programs are available at the workplace or in his community.

Standard of Practice 4.2.5

Holistic nurses promote social networks and social environments where healing can take place.

This Standard relates to healing the environment on both a personal and a professional level. All nurses have a responsibility to create a positive environment for self and others—that is, an environment free of stress to allow for peace and harmony; an environment where healing can take place. Nurses must work to minimize or completely remove stress in their work and home environments. This also means that nurses must be considerate of others and unselfish in their desires to complete their tasks. Nurses should avoid placing any undue demands on others as well as self. In relation to being a caregiver, nurses must assist clients to discover the stress that exists in their lives so that the effect of this stress can be reduced or eliminated. By recognizing that the environment is common space that is shared by many and that one person's actions can and often do have a rippling effect on all others, nurses are in a key position to impact the outcome of all relationships.

From a professional perspective, one's personal philosophy dictates the degree of involvement one is willing to invest relative to resolving environmental issues. However, because environmental concerns are important to all individuals, it is not uncommon for nurses to actively engage in activities to protect the overall health of the planet. Moreover, from a professional perspective, nurses develop a social justice ethic. They come to understand and provide care based on knowledge from a global environmental perspective. Additionally, from a professional perspective, nurses acquire knowledge about the organizations and environments within which nursing is practiced, realizing that health care policy shapes health care systems, which determines accessibility, accountability, and affordability.

Table 4–10 illustrates the nursing knowledge and skill required for a nurse to meet Standard 4.2.5.

Table 4–10 Social Networks and Environments for Healing

Standard of Practice 4.2.5	*Key Concepts*	*Requisite Knowledge*	*Requisite Skills*
Holistic nurses promote social networks and social environments where healing can take place.	Social networks for healing.	Theory and research on the web of relationships of person, environment, relationships with others/groups; relationships with others/groups that foster a sense of belonging.	Ability to communicate and develop trusting relationships; willingness to form social and community bonds; ability to show affection.
	Social environments for healing.	Environmental education and knowledge of community well-being; knowledge of health care systems and policy as it impacts delivery of health care services.	Ability to assess exposure to social stressors; ability to understand health care systems and policy; knowledge of globalization and its effects on healing.

Nursing Activities

Nursing actions that demonstrate this Standard include: developing a social justice ethic, assessing exposure to personal environmental stress; conducting environmental surveys; seeking knowledge of or appropriate consultation to understand impact of international health care policy.

In looking at how stress impacts self and others, nurses engage in or recommend that others engage in self-reevaluation—that is, assess how one's problems affect the physical environment. The primary reason for conducting environmental surveys is to determine causative agents that alter the relationships among and between organisms and between them and all aspects, living and nonliving, of their environment. Developing a social justice ethic relates to ensuring there is a fair distribution of scarce and limited resources among all members of society. Further, it is important for the holistic nurse to have knowledge and experience with health care delivery systems and policy decisions, as they impact the health care that clients receive. For example, it is important to understand the impact of accessibility or affordability for clients who lack the knowledge or communication skills to act for themselves. It is equally important to know how to help clients achieve the care they need. To illustrate, the health care options for surgery for a poor, frail elderly person must not be denied based on his or her ability to pay, nor should services be denied to a dying child because of his or her race or nationality. Nurses must act to ensure care is provided. Likewise, an essential competency for all nurses is to have knowledge and skill related to global health care issues, including an understanding of the implications of living with transportation and information technology as these factors link all parts of the world.[16]

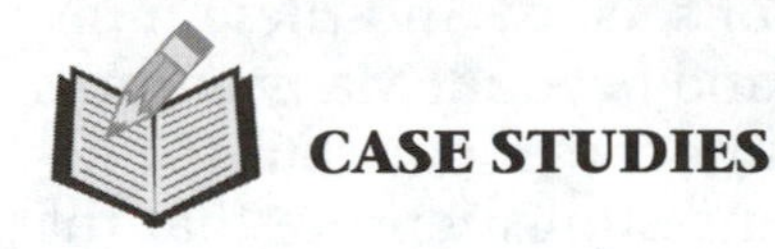

CASE STUDIES

1 Tessa is a nurse educator concerned about international law and public health policy. She became alarmed at a recent news release concerning poultry and the distribution of that food to vulnerable populations. Tessa set out to learn as much as possible about this issue with the intent of sharing all information with her students. She began to investigate how the company was handling the contaminated chickens. She wrote several letters to her congressmen and state senators for their assistance in sharing information they might have on the issue. Tessa also sought help from several concerned social groups and she accessed all available printed material from the Internet. Further, Tessa was concerned about the access people have to this country through travel. Her concern related to the fact that someone infected by contaminated foods could be a carrier of illness and could, in fact, infect someone in this country. Once all of her information was gathered, Tessa shared this information with her students, colleagues, and the community where she lives. Tessa meets Standard 4.2.5. Fortunately, as a result of Tessa being proactive related to this issue, corrective measures were required and enforced with the company handling the infected chickens to protect the public's health. Legislation to prevent similar issues in the future was passed without further debate.

2 Cooper is a registered nurse at a community health clinic. His client Nikki is being seen at the clinic for severe headaches and a skin rash. After Cooper completes a physical exam, Nikki begins to tell a story about how she believes her ex-boyfriend is stalking her. She talks of her fear in going outdoors and relates how she has remained secluded in her apartment for weeks. As she continues with her story, Cooper believes it is fabricated so he pays little attention to the remaining detail. Further, Cooper knows this client has had a mental health diagnosis in the past and suggests, through his documentation and verbal report to the primary care physician, this may indeed be happening again. He completes the exam and requests a prescription from the primary care physician for the client's skin rash.

Cooper does not meet Standard 4.2.5. He does not listen to the client's story or attempt to learn what she may have already done to resolve the problem. He does not convey an interest in the client or offer suggestions or referrals to other agencies that may help with counseling or support. Cooper did not engage the client as a partner in evolving a plan of action.

4.3 Cultural Diversity

Holistic nurses recognize each person as a whole body-mind-spirit being and mutually create a plan of care consistent with cultural background, health beliefs, sexual orientation, values, and preferences.

The concept of cultural competence is multifaceted and significantly more important today than ever before, since there is an increasing number of ethnic and racial groups who are changing the fabric of society, and these numbers are expected to grow well into the next decade and beyond. Many authors write that soon it will be difficult to tell who is a minority in our country. Regardless of which group predominates, however, nurses must ensure that the basic principles of culturally competent care are integrated into every provider's practice and in all education programs. To do this effectively, nurses must know what culturally competent care entails. It does involve asking questions about religion and racial background, as nurses have always done in the past, but effectively planned care that is culturally sensitive must also include holistic assessment data on one's life journey and how one thinks, acts, and feels. Furthermore, providing culturally sensitive care also requires nurses to recognize that culture has a tremendous influence on one's interpretation of health and illness and response to health care.

Cultural competence remains foremost on many professional agendas for other reasons as well but primarily because of the artificial barriers that exist. For example, accessibility and affordability are health care issues that create added health risks for the elderly, uninsured, and persons who are unable to care for themselves. However, many additional health problems occur because, as minority groups immigrate into the United States, many lack the ability to communicate their needs. In most clinical settings, health care providers want to provide interpreters or translators but find the funding sources are seldom seen as a priority; consequently, this needed assistance is not available. In other instances, some health care workers do not value the need to learn about the cultural values, beliefs, specific health differences, or cultural practices of the people they serve. Some believe it is the client's responsibility to adapt to the rules, regulations, and ways of the setting where they seek care. This may create potential conflicts in nurse/client relationships particularly when the response to care is evaluated as noncompliance compared to issues of response based on cultural norms or artificial barriers of accessibility. Aside from judgments made because of barriers such as accessibility, some authors point out that many nurses make value judgments and fail to provide culturally competent care because they lack self-awareness.[17] That is, nurses do not understand their own culture and its influence on one's own perceptions and behaviors. Consequently, nurses fall prey to judging individuals by how they personally respond or how they personally believe others ought to respond.

Standard of Practice 4.3.1

Holistic nurses assess and incorporate the person's cultural practices, values, beliefs, meaning of health, illness, and risk behaviors in care and health education.

This Standard underscores the nurse's responsibility to listen to a person's story. It also implies that the nurse will use reflective questioning to ensure understanding of the meaning and significance of a particular event or happening. To illustrate, a holistic nurse would base his or her care on a person's individuality and not assume he or she would respond in a particular manner typically ascribed to his or her cultural group. An example would be how a person responds to pain, which is based on past experience, not on how one should be expected to behave because of ethnic origin.

Table 4–11 illustrates the nursing knowledge and skill required for a nurse to meet Standard 4.3.1.

Table 4–11 Cultural Behavior and Health Education

Standard of Practice 4.3.1	*Key Concepts*	*Requisite Knowledge*	*Requisite Skills*
Holistic nurses assess and incorporate the person's cultural practices, values, beliefs, meaning of health, illness, and risk behaviors in care and health education.	Multifaceted influences on health.	Concepts related to cultural diversity in health and illness; concepts and models related to health traditions assessment techniques; knowledge of risk behaviors.	Ability to use cultural client assessment techniques; developing cultural competence with interventions; intercultural communication.
	Health information and education using culturally based teaching interventions.	Concepts related to self-assessment and the circle of human potential; strategies to increase ability with self-nurturing, self-care, and self-healing.	Educating persons about the relationship between lifestyle, attitudes, faith, and well-being.

Nursing Activities

Nursing actions that demonstrate this Standard include ability to conduct a cultural health assessment and ability to develop skills of communicating with someone from a different culture.

While nurses may conduct cultural assessments using several different tools, they always stress how important effective communication skills are in being able to understand one another.[1,7,17] For example, using strategies such as active listening, use of open-ended questions, and responding to a client based on what he or she deems important is common to all. Nurses who use cultural health care assessment techniques also stress the importance of refraining from cueing and leading responses. The importance of taking time to clarify, paraphrase, reflect on responses, summarize, and identify the need for validation are equally important. These many aspects of communication, however, are greatly altered when the client and the nurse have a different language. This ability to understand is also complicated when an interpreter or translator is unavailable. Yet another barrier can be how one perceives nonverbal communication. To illustrate, when people speak a different language, it is not uncommon to use hand gestures or touch when attempting to communicate, but in some cultures, gestures or touch can be perceived as inappropriate behavior. Degrees of closeness or personal space in attempting to communicate can also be misinterpreted. These issues point to the need to anticipate and be prepared in advance to deal with cultural competence issues in one's practice setting. Guidelines to deal with non-English-speaking clients or those partially fluent in English are available.[17]

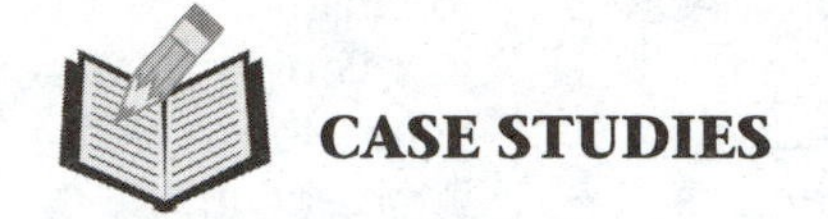

CASE STUDIES

1 Manuel is recovering from a stroke at a local rehabilitation center. He is able to communicate somewhat using eye movements, but otherwise he and his nurse Catherine are dependent on his daughter to help interpret his needs. In working with him, Catherine is able to move him about in bed, turning him on a two-hour schedule. She is very compassionate and talks to him while she is doing range of motion exercises. Since Catherine is unaware of any particular cultural beliefs about illness or rehabilitative care that are held by people of Cuban descent, she takes the time to interview Manuel's daughter during visiting hours. This action, however, has required Catherine to seek the assistance of an interpreter, since Manuel's daughter is only partially fluent in English.

Catherine's goal is to discover any particular needs Manuel may have or concerns his family may have about the various movements she does with his legs and arms. Catherine's concern is that she may be unknowingly administering care that is perceived as being too rough for an elderly man. Further, Catherine is also concerned about how Cuban families view women touching men. After her interview, Catherine learns that in the Cuban culture, elders are considered very precious and it is important to avoid any aggressive movements. Catherine adapts her care accordingly, being sure she is not exercising Manuel's extremities to a maximum that would be perceived as too hurtful. Through the interpreter, Catherine explains the need to physically move each limb in order to help Manuel regain strength and prevent contractures, with the hope of assisting Manuel to walk again in the future. Catherine meets Standard 4.3.1.

2 Pedro, a migrant worker from Mexico, was seeking care for his three-year-old son in the emergency room and was trying to explain to the nurse why the child was crying and shaking. The nurse, who saw a bruise on the child's arm, ignored the father's frantic talk and hurriedly began asking questions about the child's immunizations. She proceeded to take the child into an examining room, telling the father he could go to the waiting room and saying "The child will stop crying once you stop fretting over him."

The nurse's insensitivity may arise from a lack of understanding of cultural influences, failure to implement skills of active listening, not caring to develop a trusting relationship or understand the father's needs, or a prejudged belief that the child was abused. It could also be that this nurse believes that if Pedro wants to live in this country and receive care for himself or his family at this health care facility, he needs to follow hospital protocol. For any of these reasons, the nurse in this case example would not meet Standard 4.3.1.

Standard of Practice 4.3.2

Holistic nurses use appropriate community resources and experts to extend their understanding of different cultures.

This Standard underscores the nurse's professional responsibility to develop culturally competent skills by attempting to learn as much as possible about individuals from different cultures. This may be accomplished by calling upon others to assist in identifying the client's needs when the client is unable to convey those needs for himself or herself—for example, by using interpreters or translators. This Standard also implies that the nurse will learn culturally competent skills by engaging in continuing education courses to learn a second language or seek additional skills by attending continuing education courses within the community. This Standard could also mean that nurses are willing to support the development of neighborhood clinics where care is brought to the client within his or her own environment and where culture is automatically understood and factored into the equation of providing holistic client care. Developing culturally sensitive teaching tools or printed health care materials that are written in the client's language is critically important. Equally important is the ability to articulate an issue from another's perspective, thus recognizing and reducing resistance and defensiveness. This is particularly important when the issue involves providing care to a culturally different population. An additional aspect could be lobbying for legislation that recognizes and supports equal access and affordable care for all.

Table 4–12 illustrates the nursing knowledge and skill required for a nurse to meet Standard 4.3.2.

Table 4–12 Culture and Community Resources

Standard of Practice 4.3.2	*Key Concepts*	*Requisite Knowledge*	*Requisite Skills*
Holistic nurses use appropriate community resources and experts to extend their understanding of different cultures.	Accessing community resources.	Philosophy and practice within community agencies.	Select practice settings that implement programs based on the culturally diverse needs of clients.

continues

Table 4–12 continued

Standard of Practice 4.3.2	*Key Concepts*	*Requisite Knowledge*	*Requisite Skills*
	Cultural influences on health and illness.	Concepts related to cultural diversity, health beliefs, and values.	Engage in activities to respect, protect, and enhance a global acceptance of cultural diversity.

Nursing Activities

Nursing actions that demonstrate this Standard include: ability to be open-minded about cultural differences; ability to make referrals relative to cultural assessments; developing an awareness of one's own biases and attitudes that create barriers to direct interaction with culturally diverse groups; developing teaching and learning tools and printed materials that are culturally sensitive.

Health educators play an important role in coordinating and presenting health-related classes or courses to individuals in a way that is acceptable and sensitive to individual needs. For example, many individuals who belong to certain cultural groups are often at risk for specific illnesses, but do not receive adequate care because they do not understand how to access the health care system. Thus, it is critically important to provide health screenings for culturally diverse populations with adequate materials to explain procedures, possible findings, and appropriate follow-up care written in their own language.

To avoid appearing authoritative, it is important to focus on the concept of engagement rather than compliance in recommended behaviors. In this way, the nurse will assume less of a controlling manner and will engage the client as a partner in planning care. It is also essential that the nurse convey a respect for the client's individual healing practices, particularly when they involve alternative methods that are not congruent with traditional forms of care—or, for that matter, not consistent with the nurse's own values and beliefs.

Maintaining an awareness of and appropriately using the resources within the community is a way of bridging the gap between the client's culture and the understanding of how to effectively achieve desired client outcomes. Referring members to the most cost-effective, appropriate community health services is essential when follow-up care is required and economic constraints exist. Likewise, linking people to community resources, such as health ministries within their congregations, or assisting individuals to meet their spiritual needs must be incorporated into cultural assessment activities.

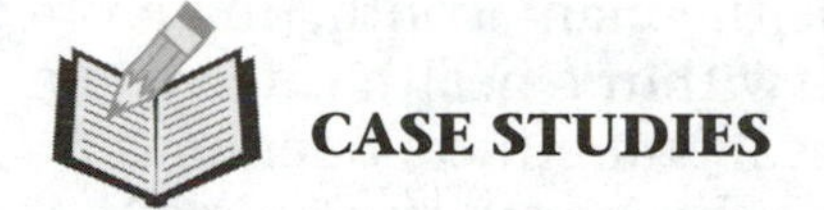

CASE STUDIES

1 Claire, a home health nurse, has recently been assigned to a neighborhood clinic in an Asian community. Her weekly visits will commence in a week, but she is worried that she will not be able to communicate effectively—not because of a language barrier, but because of her lack of knowledge about Asian customs within the home. For example, she has always heard that visitors must take off their shoes when entering Asian homes, but this practice goes against the principles she learned in public health nursing. Further, she has always been told she has a nice firm handshake, but she wonders how she should greet her clients. Does she bow as she says hello or does she shake their hands? If she shakes their hands, should it be a firm handshake, a feeble one, or simply a light touch of the palms? How does she address her clients by name? If the client is the woman but both husband and wife are in the home at the time of the visit, does she ask the client about her personal needs and care desired or will the husband make all choices?

Prior to these visits, Claire calls upon individuals within the community and asks as many questions as possible, learning as much about the Asian culture as possible to facilitate a successful visit. Claire meets Standard 4.3.2 because of her sensitive concerns and efforts to prepare herself in advance.

2 Kayla is a new clinical instructor doing prenatal visits with three students at a community health clinic. All of the clients in the clinic happen to be Hispanic women. Kayla assigns her male student to Carina, who becomes noticeably upset when he begins to palpate her abdomen to locate the appropriate area to listen to fetal heart sounds. Kayla's primary goal is to meet the student's needs; therefore, she assertively explains to Carina that this student must listen to the baby's heart sounds in order to complete his assignment. Kayla fails to talk to Carina about her concerns or to inquire why she is upset. She fails to recognize that any male (in this case a student nurse) touching a woman is not accepted in the Hispanic culture. Kayla placed the learning need of the student nurse above that of the client and failed to be sensitive to the beliefs and customs of the Hispanic women. Kayla does not meet Standard 4.3.2.

Standard of Practice 4.3.3

Holistic nurses assess for discriminatory practices and change as necessary.

Standard of Practice 4.3.4

Holistic nurses identify discriminatory health practices as they impact the person and engage in effective nondiscriminatory practices.

These two Standards dictate that nurses examine the many conflicting problems that challenge them as they attempt to work within a health care system while resolving problems that present both practical and ethical dilemmas related to client rights to care. The Standards address the many issues surrounding discriminatory practices that impact the health and well-being of individuals—of both self as practitioner and client as recipient of that care. Standard 4.3.3 relates to the work environment that obliges nurses to understand issues related to professional relationships with colleagues, institutions, and other health care workers. Standard 4.3.4 is about client care rights and the professional responsibility to provide quality care. Nurses must find solutions to problems of workplace discrimination or sexual harassment as well as resolve issues surrounding discrimination among special populations, whether the issues involve race, culture, ethnicity, age, or disability. The tables below illustrate the nursing knowledge and skill required for a nurse to meet these Standards.

Table 4–13 illustrates the nursing knowledge and skill required for a nurse to meet Standard 4.3.3.

Table 4–14 illustrates the nursing knowledge and skill required for a nurse to meet Standard 4.3.4.

Table 4–13 Discriminatory Practice in Health Care Environments

Standard of Practice 4.3.3	*Key Concepts*	*Requisite Knowledge*	*Requisite Skills*
Holistic nurses assess for discriminatory practices and change as necessary.	Discriminatory practice in health care environments.	Theory related to professional relationships; practice issues between nurses and health care systems; issues and practices concerning workplace discrimination and harassment.	Engage in decision making that supports ethical and moral principles; ability to discern loyalties; ability to resolve conflict; and ability to treat others fairly and equitably.

Table 4–14 Effective Nondiscriminatory Practice

Standard of Practice 4.3.4	*Key Concepts*	*Requisite Knowledge*	*Requisite Skills*
Holistic nurses identify discriminatory health practices as they impact the person and	Client rights/needs for professional care.	Concepts related to transcending personal beliefs and prejudices; assessing data to evaluate the client's total state of	Engage in activities to be open-minded; view the world perceptively and listen with focused intention; ability to integrate concepts

continues

Table 4–14 continued

Standard of Practice 4.3.4	*Key Concepts*	*Requisite Knowledge*	*Requisite Skills*
engage in effective nondiscriminatory practices.		being/elements that give meaning to a person's life.	of whole client care including the therapeutic use of self.
	Effective non-discriminatory practice.	Standards of care related to shared humanness including a sense of being connected to and attentive to clients as unique persons.	Implement professional practice guided by a holistic framework; ability to recognize each person as a unique being worthy of respect.

Nursing Activities

Nursing actions that demonstrate these Standards include ability to: examine personal values and beliefs, respect persons as unique individuals, make decisions that support ethical and moral principles, prioritize obligations, examine differences in loyalties, respect diverse opinions, review skills of negotiation, and maintain relationships guided by the professional code of ethics.

Examining personal values and beliefs relates to the nurse's ability to problem-solve and make decisions about maintaining client welfare while at the same time dealing with problems among other providers and within institutions. The nurse enters the workforce and progresses from novice to expert in developing his or her technical and professional skills. Often, however, the nurse is forced to come to terms with practice issues that in his/her opinion compromise quality care—for example, staffing problems requiring larger numbers of clients per nurse or the nurse being floated to another department where he or she is unprepared to provide the same degree of quality care. In some instances, the practice issue creates a conflict in meeting the nurse's self-care needs and the system's expectation of loyalty, which is viewed as inequitable and creates professional dilemmas that often result in the nurse leaving his or her job. Some problems surround issues of sexual harassment or discrimination where power and coercion impact relationships. Yet in other situations the discrimination relates to special populations of individuals with special care needs who are at increased risk for varied health problems, illness, or disease. The discrimination could be aimed at cultural or ethnic groups; however, age and disability often cause conflicts to surface where the practice issue for nurses relates to who receives the health care services and the quality of the service that is provided.

Respecting persons as unique individuals relates to the nurse's ability to recognize that person as an autonomous being worthy of respect and care. Nurses must provide services to anyone regardless of national origin, race, age, sex, or disability. Yet a nurse may witness discrimination and think of him or herself as powerless to change the situation. Even more alarming is the situation of blind loyalty to another nurse or health care provider. In protecting an incompetent coworker who practices inadequately or inappropriately or who abuses or neglects clients, the nurse who fails to report another, either because of misguided or fanatical loyalty, is equally accountable for harming the client and failing to integrate the principle of beneficence (doing good for another).

In the Standards regarding discrimination surrounding a nurse's practice, and particularly for issues linked to bottom-line economics within the health care system, nurses are required to address issues of change. In the workplace, a nurse expects his or her opinion related to practice issues to be valued and respected but often finds there are as many varied opinions and ways of doing as there are differing groups of people. Therefore, a certain amount of conformity is necessary when working with others, and nurses must reach consensus in resolving practice issues. Additionally, a nurse must often articulate an issue from the perspective of recognizing and reducing his or her defensiveness. While many struggle to keep certain core values, beliefs, and traditions in place, change requires that uniformity and sameness yield to a combination of ways, and thus a new fabric is woven. Examples relating to such changes can be seen in acute care settings where nurses are being asked to do more with less, to supervise unlicensed personnel, or to be creative in designing new approaches to providing care for clients.

CASE STUDIES

1 Nurse Alexis and nurse Maggie held similar views with respect to how nursing should be practiced on their unit. Both had practiced using a functional model of care delivery for over 15 years and were unbending when it came to change. They also held similar views with respect to who the health care provider ought to be and how that person ought to be trained. They both considered themselves to be excellent nurses and they wanted to remain bedside nurses responsible for the nursing activities that were now being delegated to unlicensed assistive personnel. Alexis and Maggie resisted the managerial responsibilities that were now being assigned to them. They did not support the development of new documentation systems, and they felt the new clinical pathway tools were too complex and failed to address individual client needs. When asked to float to other units when staffing shortages existed, they refused. They found they disagreed with the hospital's request to have staff work additional hours when budget cuts necessitated fewer employees even though

the same amount of work was needed to meet client needs. Their loyalty to the institution was being challenged, and they faced daily dilemmas with respect to how to deliver client care.

Eventually, both Alexis and Maggie returned to school to earn their baccalaureate degrees. Soon after they registered for the nursing issues course, they found themselves embroiled in arguments relating to the seemingly small amount of time the BSN student spends on gaining technical skills. They quickly voiced their opinion on many issues, showing they were not open to new ideas or ways of doing. The course required both students to read in depth and to engage in debates about practice issues. Their views were challenged and they were obliged to listen to others. Both were required to develop change projects, and in that assignment it became evident to them how resistive they had been. During one class session, Alexis conceded that she believed all nurses ought to practice as she did. Now she saw many unique perspectives. She said, "It is like getting a new pair of glasses and seeing points of view that I never saw before." Maggie made a similar statement as she professed that nurse-client relationships were not negatively impacted—rather, she now believed the new hospital arrangements really did improve quality of care to clients. Both Alexis and Maggie meet Standard 4.3.3.

2 Sam, a registered nurse, works on a skilled nursing unit that has many residents who have been diagnosed with Alzheimer's disease and who are in varying stages of debilitation. Staff shortages are a common occurrence and many employees call in sick without apparent regard for the residents' welfare. Sam, overwhelmed by his responsibilities, works tirelessly to provide care, missing his dinner often and working extra hours to complete all his required written documentation. He reports his increased workload responsibilities to his supervisor but notes that change does not appear to be forthcoming. No additional staff have been hired and temporary staff are not utilized. Yet, remaining loyal to his employer, Sam continues to accept this burden.

As the weeks pass, Sam finds that his ability to provide all of the treatments as ordered is becoming more and more difficult. On some days, skin care is not given as often as ordered and medications are administered late. Some of the required care related to walking residents and engaging them in diversional activities is simply not done. Further, individual residents are not being supervised in the dining area and many are not eating properly. Edith, one of the residents, has very edematous feet and she is often incontinent, requiring more frequent attention for toileting. Additionally, she has quite a noticeable deterioration of cognitive ability along with being very unstable on her feet. She has fallen several times and has several bruise marks on the side of her face and both arms. Consequently, she is restrained and not walked as often as required. When her sister Alice calls to inquire of her condition, Sam reports that she is maintaining her own and being cared for in the best possible way. Sam is torn when he reports on Edith's physical condition. He knows he is not being truthful with reports to her sister and that, indeed, her condition is deteriorating more quickly than if proper care were being provided. Sam believes Alice has the right to know of Edith's condition but fails to report it to her, believing that it could result in his being disciplined for failing to provide adequate and proper care related to acts of omission. He further believes that he could lose his job if he reports his employer or, still worse, be implicated in a lawsuit for neglect and abuse.

Sam does not meet Standard 3.4.4. While he is providing the best possible care under the conditions of his current employment, he takes no action to resolve the dilemmas other than to report the work strain to his supervisor. Sam does not examine the associated ethical dilemmas of his work situation, nor does he investigate the possible harm that could result to other residents if the issues surrounding adequate staffing are not addressed in this setting.

CONCLUSION

The foundational concepts essential for holistic nurses, communication, therapeutic environment, and cultural diversity are presented in Core Value 4 through a myriad of nursing activities that, when performed, demonstrate practice that is consistent with the Standards of Care and the Standards of Practice.

Communication is the basis of the nurse/client/family relationship and among the most critical components to ensure the caring and healing of clients. Sharing an authentic and sincere experience, by learning the art of "listening," is clearly viewed as an inherent goal to establishing a therapeutic nurse-client interaction. Communication, a valued concept within the nurse's practice setting, is viewed as a critical component to establishing professional work relationships with others. Using techniques such as focused exploration and active problem solving are ways holistic nurses can identify, diminish, and/or eliminate the barriers to effective communication. Facilitating communication, from the perspective of providing culturally competent care, is presented from the viewpoint of its influence on client outcomes. Understanding and accepting the cultural beliefs, values, and practices of the ethnic origins of others is discussed from the standpoint of the nurse's ability to develop a self awareness by effectively listening to his or her beliefs and recognizing they are not common to all. The role of the nurse in helping the client to find meaning and purpose in life, illness, suffering, or challenge is presented from the approach of being fully present and developing an inner strength and connectedness with self, others, nature, and God/Life Force/Absolute Transcendent. Lastly, recognizing that communication is a continuously evolving, multilevel exchange within all relationships, the value of caring for the mind/body/spirit with the use of interventions such as relaxation and imagery were presented. Critically important, as the last theme of communication, was the responsibility to accept the client's ability to identify his or her own alternate ways of knowing and choosing.

Therapeutic environment was presented from the perspective of its internal and external influence on client health and well-being. An equally important concept within the Standards of Care is the ability to provide for sacred space in recognition of the client's need for quiet, personal prayer or meditation. Understanding the relationship of health to the natural world and the ways in which diseases are related to, or caused by something in the environment, is viewed as fundamental concepts required to effectively practice holistic nursing. The nurse's responsibility to be personally active in maintaining environmental quality is seen as important as stressing this need to one's clients/families/communities. In the end, the holistic nurse demonstrates accountability to promote health, facilitate healing, and alleviate suffering by providing healing environments, supporting professional networks and social environments, and developing a commitment to lifelong learning.

Ways to enhance cultural sensitivity and cultural competence in holistic practice are viewed as critically important concepts rooted in individual diversity and differences in health practices. Cultural health assessments and planning client care that incorporates values, beliefs, and customs are vital for reducing or eliminating at-risk behaviors. Using referrals or calling on the expertise of others to learn of the ways of persons from different cultures is evidence of being professionally accountable. Taking action to eliminate discriminatory health practices is presented as one of the last nursing actions in holistic practice for Core Value 4.

NOTES

1. B.M. Dossey et al., *Holistic Nursing: A Handbook for Practice*, 3d ed. (Gaithersburg, MD: Aspen Publishers, 1999).
2. S. Scandrett-Hibdon, "Therapeutic Communication: The Art of Helping," in *American Holistic Nurses' Association Core Curriculum for Holistic Nursing*, ed. B.M. Dossey (Gaithersburg, MD: Aspen Publishers, 1997), 102–107.
3. J. Engebretson, "Cultural Diversity and Care," in *American Holistic Nurses' Association Core Curriculum for Holistic Nursing*, ed. B.M. Dossey (Gaithersburg, MD: Aspen Publishers, 1997), 108–118.
4. L.C. Callistere et al., "Cultural and Spiritual Meanings of Childbirth," *Journal of Holistic Nursing* 17, no. 3 (1999): 280–295.
5. M.A. Burkhardt, "Becoming and Connecting: Elements of Spirituality for Women," in *Essential Readings in Holistic Nursing*, ed. C.E. Guzzetta (Gaithersburg, MD: Aspen Publishers, 1998), 46–54.
6. J. Walton, "Spirituality of Patients Recovering from an Acute Myocardial Infarction," *Journal of Holistic Nursing* 17, no. 1 (1999): 34–53.
7. J.B. Riley, *Communication in Nursing* (St. Louis: Mosby, 2000), 219–233.
8. V. Andrus and J.Y. Lunt, "Bringing Holistic Nursing into the New Millennium," *Alternative and Complementary Therapies* (February 1987): 24–28.
9. B.M. Dossey, "Imagery," in *American Holistic Nurses' Association Core Curriculum for Holistic Nursing*, ed. B.M. Dossey (Gaithersburg, MD: Aspen Publishers, 1997), 188–195.
10. B.L. Rees, "An Exploratory Study of the Effectiveness of a Relaxation with Guided Imagery Protocol," *Journal of Holistic Nursing* 11, no. 3 (1993): 271–276.
11. D.J. Bazzo and R.A. Moeller, "Imagine This! Infinite Uses of Guided Imagery in Women's Health," *Journal of Holistic Nursing* 17, no. 4 (1999): 317–330.
12. B.M. Dossey et al., *The Art Of Caring* (Boulder, CO: Sounds True, 1996).
13. E.A. Schuster, "Environment," in *American Holistic Nurses' Association Core Curriculum for Holistic Nursing*, ed. B.M. Dossey (Gaithersburg, MD: Aspen Publishers, 1997), 164–169.
14. J.F. Quinn, "Holding Sacred Space," in *Essential Readings in Holistic Nursing*, ed. C.E. Guzzetta (Gaithersburg, MD: Aspen Publishers, 1998), 84–93.

15. B. Johnson, "Holistic Nursing: A Breed of Its Own," in *Tennessee Nurse* 62, no. 1 (1999): 11–17.
16. L. Acord, Chairperson of Task Force, *The Essentials of Baccalaureate Education*, American Association of Colleges of Nursing (Washington, DC, 1998).
17. M.A. Burkhardt and A.K. Nathaniel, *Ethics & Issues in Contemporary Nursing* (Albany, NY: Delmar Publishers, 1998), 318–324.

CORE VALUE 5

HOLISTIC CARING PROCESS

Cathie E. Guzzetta

The holistic caring process is a circular process that involves six steps, which may occur simultaneously. These parts are assessment, pattern/problems/needs, outcomes, therapeutic care plan, implementation, and evaluation.

The holistic caring process, as the fifth Core Value, is an adaptation of the nursing process that integrates holistic philosophy. It is a circular process, focusing on the establishment of health and well-being of the client, that includes six steps: assessment, patterns/problems/needs, outcomes, therapeutic care plan, implementation, and evaluation. Expert nurses realize, however, that the six steps are rarely executed in a linear sequence. During the first encounter with a client, the nurse is simultaneously assessing, diagnosing, and evaluating. Likewise, the nurse's presence, caring, and listening during the encounter provide immediate caring interventions which are continuously evaluated.[1]

The holistic caring process is an organized, ongoing, living framework for discovering, describing, and documenting health patterns unique to each person. These patterns, identified within the nurse-person relationship, provide the information by which to establish common outcomes, select and implement appropriate interventions, and evaluate responses to actions initiated within the holistic caring process.[2]

The holistic caring process is guided by holistic nursing philosophy embedded within a conceptual model of nursing that unifies, standardizes, and directs nursing practice. The process is interactive, interpersonal, and client-centered.[3] The client (rather than the disease) is viewed as the primary focus of the nurse-client relationship in which the unique bio-psycho-social-spiritual dimensions of the whole person are addressed. By incorporating both the problem-solving components of natural science methodology and the caring dimension of the human science approach, the client's realities, perceptions, and life meanings are incorporated into the holistic caring process to individualize the client's lived experience of health, illness, and well-being.[2]

The client is viewed as a participant in identifying and pursuing outcomes for health care. Thus, the client assumes as active a role as possible in health care assessment and decision making about patterns/problems/needs, outcomes, planning, interventions, and evaluation in order to take responsibility for personal health care choices and decisions for self-care.

5.1 ASSESSMENT

■■ Each person is assessed holistically using appropriate traditional and holistic methods while the uniqueness of the person is honored. ■■

Assessment is the information-gathering phase of the holistic caring process. The nurse, in collaboration with the client, identifies health patterns and prioritizes the health care concerns. Assessment is an ongoing process providing for continuous collection of data so that changes in the client's health status can be evaluated over time. Thus, each nurse-client encounter furnishes new information by which to interpret patterns and interrelationships and verifies previous inferences and conclusions. Two Standards of Practice demonstrate the Core Value of assessment, as described and illustrated below.

Standard of Practice 5.1.1

Holistic nurses use an assessment process including appropriate traditional and holistic methods to systematically gather information.

Standard of Practice 5.1.2

Holistic nurses value all types of knowing including intuition when gathering data from a person and validate this intuitive knowledge with the person when appropriate.

These Standards emphasize the Core Value that holistic nurses place on conducting a bio-psycho-social-spiritual assessment of the client. Performing a holistic assessment demands clustering and synthesizing the subjective and objective data that reflect the client's bio-psycho-social-spiritual responses to health and illness. In doing so, it is critical that the appropriate data be collected and evaluated. Holistic nurses therefore collect data to evaluate information about the client's patterns by using traditional history and physical examination approaches as well as by objective measurements that provide quantifiable information obtained from instruments, monitors, and laboratory data to identify human response patterns and deviations. Information is also gathered through an assessment of the client's energy fields as well as through client interactions, observations gleaned from the five senses, and intuitive perceptions to uncover subtle attitudes, values, feelings, and thoughts about health and illness patterns as understood only by the client. Holistic nurses value equally data obtained from qualitative and quantitative approaches to assessment. As patterns are recognized, each becomes a hologram of the person, contributing to an understanding of the whole.

Assessment and documentation of the patterns are ongoing, because changes in one pattern always influence the other dimensions. Holistic nurses are also aware of their own personal values, beliefs, and patterns—especially related to differences in culture, socioeconomic class, age, gender, sexual orientation, education, or physical limitations—and their effects on the collection and interpretation of data.[2]

Table 5–1 illustrates the nursing knowledge and skills required for a nurse to meet Standards 5.1.1 and 5.1.2.

Table 5–1 Nursing Knowledge and Skills in Holistic Assessment

Standard of Practice 5.1.1	*Key Concepts*	*Requisite Knowledge*	*Requisite Skills*
Holistic nurses use an assessment process including appropriate traditional and holistic methods to systematically gather information.	Traditional assessment skills. Holistic assessment skills. Systematically gathering information.	Knowledge of human response patterns and deviations. Knowledge of traditional health history and physical examination skills. Knowledge of quantifiable, objective data. Knowledge of holistic assessment skills to assess bio-psycho-social-spiritual patterns using interactions, observations, intuition, energy fields. Recognizing personal values, beliefs, and patterns.	Willingness to participate with patient in assessment. Centeredness. Intention. Presence. Listening. Interviewing and physical assessment skills (inspection, palpation, percussion, auscultation). Interpersonal therapeutic communication skills. Ability to collect, organize, and synthesize complex data. Using inductive/deductive reasoning skills.
Standard of Practice 5.1.2	*Key Concepts*	*Requisite Knowledge*	*Requisite Skills*
Holistic nurses value all types of knowing including intuition when gathering data from a person and validate this intuitive knowledge with the person when appropriate.	Ways of knowing. Intuition. Client validation.	Valuing right and left brain thinking. Valuing intuitive knowledge. Valuing importance of client's validation and meaning of health care concerns.	Willingness to partner with client. Clinical reasoning. Intuitive thinking.

Nursing Activities

The holistic caring process begins with the first moment of client contact.[3] It also begins "where the client is" by asking the client (and family/significant others) to share information that will identify the client's primary reasons for seeking help, inviting a complete articulation of their concerns, worries, and fears.[1,3] Thus, the client is encouraged to fully participate with the nurse in the data-gathering process.

Before entering into the nurse-client encounter, holistic nurses make every effort to become centered or balanced to allow optimum levels of attention and presence to the moment.[4] They also enter into the nurse-client encounter with intention, which involves the awareness of creating an image of a person's spiritual essence and their wholeness experienced as a "sacred space."[4] In addition, the encounter necessitates that the nurse be fully present. Such nursing presence contains a relational style and quality of "being with" and "collaborating with" rather than "doing to" the client.[4,5] "Being with" implies a conscious intention to appreciate the shared experience of the "now" in which the nurse confronts the uncertainties of the situation, goes beyond the objective data to understand subtle and intricate cues to sense the whole of the situation, and connects with the client's experiences.[6] Nursing presence is both an acquired skill used to accomplish a holistic assessment and an intervention that can release a response from an individual that can bring perspective, discernment, alignment, balance, meaning, well-being, and healing.[7]

Performing a holistic assessment demands a mindful process that is deliberate and attentive in gathering the appropriate data by which to assess the patient's bio-psycho-social-spiritual patterns/problems/needs. Unfortunately, in many hospitals and health care institutions and clinics, nurses gather and cluster data around the traditional medical database that focuses on disease. Such traditional databases include information about the patient's past medical history, a review of systems, a physical examination (using inspection, palpation, percussion, and auscultation), and data gathered about some psychosocial questions that have been arbitrarily added to the beginning or end of the assessment form. Yet the use of a traditional medical database does not permit a holistic assessment to emerge, because the patient is assessed primarily from a medical point of view. As a result, only part of the data is collected with which to assess the whole patient.[8]

To accomplish a holistic assessment, some type of holistic framework, model, or classification system must be used to guide the collection of data to ensure an assessment of the whole person. Many of the holistic theories discussed in Core Value 2.2 can be used to develop the structure and terminology of a holistic database. Such theories help identify the assessment variables that should be included in the holistic database and provide the structure necessary to understand how the data are interrelated and organized to uncover patterns that reveal meaningful wholes. Other frameworks that can be used for assessing the whole person include the North American Nursing Diagnosis

Association's (NANDA's) nine human response patterns[9] (Exhibit 5–1). Using this framework, relevant data are clustered and collected to assess each of these nine patterns to achieve a holistic assessment. Examples of this tool for use with hospitalized patients or with clients in a wellness or health care clinic setting are given in Appendixes 5-A and 5-B. Likewise, Gordon's eleven functional health patterns[10] have been used to develop a format for patient assessment and as a guide by which to organize data (Exhibit 5–2).

Exhibit 5–1 Nine Human Response Patterns

1. Exchanging: a human response pattern involving mutual giving and receiving
2. Communicating: a human response pattern involving sending messages
3. Relating: a human response pattern involving establishing bonds
4. Valuing: a human response pattern involving the assigning of relative worth
5. Choosing: a human response pattern involving the selection of alternatives
6. Moving: a human response pattern involving activity
7. Perceiving: a human response pattern involving the reception of information
8. Knowing: a human response pattern involving the meaning associated with information
9. Feeling: a human response pattern involving subjective awareness of information

Source: Reprinted with permission from C. Roy, Framework for Classification Systems Development: Progress and Issues, in *Classification of Nursing Diagnoses: Proceedings of the Fifth Conference*, M.J. Kim et al., eds., pp. 40–45, © 1984, Mosby-Year Book, Inc.

Exhibit 5–2 Typology of Gordon's Functional Health Patterns

1. *Health perception–health management pattern:* perceptions about one's health and how those perceptions shape personal health practices
2. *Nutritional–metabolic pattern:* one's biopsychosocial status in relation to the food and water supply and to nutrient and food intake
3. *Elimination pattern:* relates to elimination through the gastrointestinal tract, urinary tract, and skin
4. *Activity–exercise pattern:* motivation and capability to engage in energy-consuming activities
5. *Sleep–rest pattern:* one's perceptions of rest and sleep practices
6. *Cognitive–perceptual pattern:* one's ability to perceive, understand, remember, make decisions, and process information from both the internal and external environment
7. *Self-perception:* one's attitudes toward self and self-competency

continues

Exhibit 5–2 continued

8. *Role–relationship pattern:* one's need for and actual interactions with others (e.g., co-workers, family, community)
9. *Sexuality–reproductive pattern:* one's actual and perceived satisfaction or dysfunction in sexuality or reproduction
10. *Coping–stress intolerance pattern:* one's adaptive or maladaptive responses to stress and change
11. *Value–belief pattern:* one's beliefs and values guiding life choices and lifestyle

Source: Reprinted with permission from G.K. McFarland and E.A. McFarland, *Nursing Diagnosis & Intervention: Planning for Patient Care,* © 1993, Mosby-Year Book, Inc.

Holistic assessment of the patient involves gathering of data not only from a rational, logical, analytic (or left-brain) mode but also from an intuitive, nonverbal (right-brain) mode.[2] Information gained from intuitive perceptions allows one to know more than he or she can explain. It is another dimension of knowing things and events without the conscious use of rational processes.[4,11] Clinical intuition is a "process by which we know something about a patient which cannot be verbalized or is verbalized poorly or for which the source of the knowledge cannot be determined."[12] It is a gut feeling that something has changed, that something is wrong, or that we should do something, even if there is no real evidence to support the feeling.[2] Intuitive thinking is facilitated by experience; direct contact with the patient; being open, emotionally able, and receptive to cues and feelings occurring; and feeling confident about the information received and the situations that warrant immediate action.[11,12] Holistic nurses also highly value the client's intuitive perceptions about how they are feeling or how things have changed, because they recognize that the client is often the first to know when something is different.[13]

The holistic nurse views clients as a whole and listens for their story and the meaning that the current health situation holds for them. When a client wants help with a specific physical problem, such as chronic pain related to arthritis, the nurse gathers the appropriate data, which are then shared and validated with the client, to establish a baseline assessment. Family/significant others, other health care providers, previous health care information, and measurable data contribute supplemental information. The client, however, is the primary source and interpreter of the meaning of the data that are obtained from the holistic assessment. In collaboration with the client, the nurse shares with the client the synthesized data and the patterns recognized from the assessment. The client then verifies the existence of the pattern and its meaning so that interventions can be selected collaboratively that are safe and acceptable to the client, and reevaluated with the client to determine if outcomes have been achieved.[3] The results of the assessment are documented in the client's record for the purposes of communicating the client's status and collaborating with other members of the health care team.

CASE STUDIES

1 Mrs. C.Z., an 80-year-old woman, was brought into the emergency room by her husband, for a severe leg laceration sustained after a fall at home. Her husband, a retired family practice physician, was very anxious about the severity of her laceration and believed his wife needed an immediate skin graft. Nurse Larry took Mrs. Z.'s vital signs and assessed the laceration and Mrs. Z.'s associated pain. Mrs. Z. was alert and oriented but clearly restless and stated she was in discomfort. She also complained of nausea but denied any recent vomiting, diarrhea, or loss of consciousness.

Larry probed further into the circumstances concerning the fall. Mrs. Z. stated she had fallen three times in the past two years but always because she tripped on some object in her way. She revealed that this fall was different and described it as if her "muscles weren't working." Larry felt the need to probe further. Mrs. Z. finally admitted that she had fallen a total of five times that day but did not believe that information was important since she had not received any injuries from the first four falls. Larry shared his uneasiness about the reasons for the multiple falls with the patient and husband. He reassured Mrs. Z. with a gentle touch that he would return with medication to help her pain. Larry immediately contacted the surgeon on call to report his findings and his concerns about possible bone fractures and head trauma (although the assessment findings revealed that the patient was neurologically stable) related to the fall as well as his suspicions about an electrolyte abnormality.

Larry returned to the room and administered a mild pain medication to the patient, suggesting to Mrs. Z. that she practice some slow, diaphragmatic breathing. He sat at the bedside holding Mrs. Z.'s hand and asked her to imagine the pain medication circulating throughout her body, feeling the warmth and comfort of the medication working in her bloodstream, and "seeing" the pain medication going directly to her leg to ease her discomfort. He then explained to her that the physician had ordered a head CT, plain X-rays of the chest and cervical spine, and laboratory work. He patiently answered the husband's medical questions and assured them both that he would continue to be with them during this assessment period to assist them with their needs and answer their questions.

Mrs. Z.'s husband remained at the bedside and accompanied his wife to each of her tests. Within a few hours, the results of the radiographic studies, which were found to be negative, were shared with the patient and husband. At this time, the patient was resting comfortably. However, it was disclosed to them that Mrs. Z.'s serum sodium, found to be 119 mmol/L indicating severe acute symptomatic hyponatremia, needed to be treated urgently with saline and was likely the reason that her "muscles were not working." The patient and husband agreed that plans for treating her laceration with a skin graft should be postponed and she should be immediately hospitalized.

Larry is practicing Standards 5.1.1 and 5.1.2 that support traditional and holistic approaches of assessment. His presence relates a conscious intention to be present in the "now" of the patient's experience. He recognizes that the patient's husband is an integral and comforting dimension in the patient's life and facilitates his presence throughout the assessment period. He recognizes the patient's acute pain and implements relaxation and imagery strategies to enhance the effects of the pain medication. In addition, Larry has a gut feeling that there is more to the story about the patient's current fall than is being revealed. He chooses to confront the uncertainties of the situation, goes beyond the limited facts available, and tries to sense the whole of the situation. In doing so, he values and trusts his intuitive hunches about the patient's condition, probes further into the patient's experience, and is confident in both acting upon and reporting this information to expedite action. The severe leg laceration, which was the central focus of the emergency room visit, in fact did warrant a skin graft, but it became a secondary problem to the immediate need of treating Mrs. Z.'s severe hyponatremia.

2 Nurse Angela was working in the emergency department when Mr. R., 66 years old, was brought in with the chief complaint of chest pain. Angela questioned Mr. R. about his pattern of pain. The patient related that the pain started about six months ago, was usually brought on by exertion, and was relieved by rest. Over the past two days, however, the episodes of pain had increased even while resting in a chair.

The patient denied any ankle edema, nocturnal dyspnea, or orthopnea. He stated that his father had died of a heart attack at age 67. Upon physical assessment, Angela found that the patient's vital signs, respiratory exam, and heart sounds were all normal (without an S3, S4, or murmurs). She determined that the patient was in normal sinus rhythm without ectopy and that his ECG and preliminary cardiac enzymes also were normal.

Following the cardiologist's consultation and recommendation that Mr. R. be hospitalized for observation, Angela administered the order for aspirin. She described how it worked and explained that it was being given based on Mr. R.'s suspected underlying heart disease. Although she reinforced that his symptoms warranted further observation and evaluation, she reassured the patient that the findings of his preliminary examination were "good news" because no heart damage had been found.

Angela's astute history taking and physical assessment skills are consistent with proficient emergency room practice. Her actions are deliberate, seasoned, and swift. She reassures the patient of his condition, answers his questions, and teaches him about his medical treatment and ongoing plan of care. Angela's actions are not consistent with Holistic Standards 5.1.1 and 5.1.2, however, because she makes no effort to connect with the patient's experience. Her relational style is one of "doing to" rather than "being with" the patient. She makes no attempts to uncover his concerns, worries, or fears related to the similarities of his history to that of his father who died, at age 67, of a myocardial infarction. There is nothing in Angela's assessment that seeks to discover current stressors in his life and daily activities that may be associated with the recent acceleration of his angina. Moreover, she does not explore with the patient his own intuitive insight about how he feels or why he believes things have changed over the past few days. In short, Angela has not succeeded in uncovering the patient's story and the meaning that the current situation holds for him.

5.2 Patterns/Problems/Needs

■■ ***Each person's actual and potential patterns/problems/needs and life processes related to health, wellness, disease, or illness that may or may not facilitate well-being are identified and prioritized.*** ■■

Following a bio-psycho-social-spiritual assessment of the client, the data are clustered, synthesized, evaluated, and interpreted. Using critical and intuitive thinking and application of theory, the client's patterns/problems/needs and life processes are identified, prioritized, and documented so that desired outcomes and a plan of care can be mutually formulated. There are four Standards of Practice that demonstrate the Core Value related to identifying patterns/problems/needs and life processes, as described and illustrated below.

Standard of Practice 5.2.1

Holistic nurses assist the person to access inner wisdom that can provide opportunities to enhance and support growth, development, and movement toward health and well-being.

Standard of Practice 5.2.2

Holistic nurses collect data and collaborate with the person and health care team members as appropriate to identify and record a list of actual and potential patterns/problems/needs.

Standard of Practice 5.2.3

Holistic nurses use collected data to formulate an etiology of the person's identified actual or potential patterns/problems/needs.

Standard of Practice 5.2.4

Holistic nurses make referrals to other holistic practitioners or traditional therapist when appropriate.

These Standards emphasize that holistic nurses value and recognize the individual's own inherent capacity for body-mind-spirit healing. The Standards dictate that nurses assist clients to access this inner wisdom. In doing so, holistic nurses provide opportunities to enhance an individual's innate abilities for growth, development, health, and well-being. In addition, the nursing role of identifying the client's actual or potential patterns/problems/needs and life processes and their causes or related factors is clearly delineated. Depending on the pattern/problem/need, the Standards also underscore the need to make referrals to both conventional and holistic practitioners as appropriate.

Table 5–2 illustrates the nursing knowledge and skills required for a nurse to meet Standards 5.2.1, 5.2.2, 5.2.3, and 5.2.4.

Table 5–2 Nursing Knowledge and Skills in Identifying Patterns/Problems/Needs

Standard of Practice 5.2.1	*Key Concepts*	*Requisite Knowledge*	*Requisite Skills*
Holistic nurses assist the person to access inner wisdom that can provide opportunities to enhance and support growth, development, and movement toward health and well-being.	Assist client to access inner wisdom. Provide opportunities to enhance and support. Growth. Development. Health. Well-being.	Knowledge of body-mind healing. Knowledge of bio-psycho-social-spiritual growth and development. Understanding dimensions of health and well-being.	Ability to recognize the client's inherent ability for self-healing. Expertise in providing opportunities to enhance and support client in the movement toward health and well-being.
Standard of Practice 5.2.2	*Key Concepts*	*Requisite Knowledge*	*Requisite Skills*
Holistic nurses collect data and collaborate with the person and health care team members as appropriate to identify and record a list of actual and potential patterns/problem/needs.	Collect data. Collaborate with client and health care team members. Identify and document patterns/problems/needs.	Knowledge of human response patterns and deviations. Knowledge of standardized nursing diagnoses terminology. Knowledge of defining characteristics, observable cues, and inferences for diagnoses.	Proficiency in clustering, synthesizing, evaluating, and interpreting data. Ability to identify actual, risk, and wellness diagnoses. Experience in validating with client existence and meaning of diagnosis. Skills in prioritizing diagnoses with client. Documentation of prioritized diagnoses.

continues

Table 5–2 continued

Standard of Practice 5.2.3	*Key Concepts*	*Requisite Knowledge*	*Requisite Skills*
Holistic nurses use collected data to formulate an etiology of the person's identified actual or potential patterns/problems/ needs.	Use data collected. Formulate etiology of pattern/ problem/need.	Knowledge of related factors causing or associated with, related to, or abetting an actual problem. Knowledge of risk factors that contribute to increased vulnerability.	Ability to determine the etiology or related factors associated with an actual diagnosis and validate with client. Ability to determine the risk factors that place a client at risk for developing a risk diagnosis and validate with client.

Standard of Practice 5.2.4	*Key Concepts*	*Requisite Knowledge*	*Requisite Skills*
Holistic nurses make referrals to other holistic practitioners or traditional therapist when appropriate.	Make referrals to holistic practitioners. Make referrals to conventional therapists.	Knowledge of various holistic and conventional health care provider roles. Knowledge of need for referrals.	Skills in referring client to reliable holistic and conventional practitioners based on client's pattern/problem/ needs. Ability to validate with client need and importance for referral.

Nursing Activities

The Standards within the second step of the holistic caring process direct nurses to identify a client's patterns/problems/needs and life processes based on standardized language that can be communicated to nurses, other health care clinicians, and managed care providers as well as to the client receiving the care. NANDA's nursing diagnoses provide the language to communicate common patterns identified by nurses across subspecialty practice. NANDA has defined a nursing diagnosis as a "clinical judgment about the individual, family, or community responses to actual and potential health problems/life processes. Nursing diagnoses provide the basis for selection of nursing interventions to achieve outcomes for which the nurse is accountable."[9]

NANDA's nursing diagnoses (Exhibit 5–3), classified according to the nine human response patterns (Exhibit 5–1), are divided into three categories: actual diagnoses, risk diagnoses, and wellness nursing diagnoses. An actual nursing diagnosis describes "human responses to health conditions/life processes that exist in an individual, family, or community."[9] In formulating an actual nursing diagnosis, health problems are labeled in terms of a pattern of related cues (e.g., energy field disturbances related to slowing or blocking of energy because of recent surgery). The related factors are those components that are associated with some type of patterned relationship to the nursing diagnosis. Related factors may be the cause of, antecedent to, associated with, related to, or abetting the problem.[9] Because they help to determine what is preventing improvement toward health, related factors help to direct the plan of care by indicating changes that are necessary to move the client toward health.

Exhibit 5–3 NANDA-Approved Nursing Diagnoses

This list represents the NANDA-approved nursing diagnoses for clinical use and testing.

Pattern 1: Exchanging

1.1.2.1	Altered Nutrition: More Than Body Requirements
1.1.2.2	Altered Nutrition: Less Than Body Requirements
1.1.2.3	Altered Nutrition: Risk for More Than Body Requirements
1.2.1.1	Risk for Infection
1.2.2.1	Risk for Altered Body Temperature
1.2.2.2	Hypothermia
1.2.2.3	Hyperthermia
1.2.2.4	Ineffective Thermoregulation
1.2.3.1	Dysreflexia
1.2.3.2	Risk for Autonomic Dysreflexia
1.3.1.1	Constipation
1.3.1.1.1	Perceived Constipation
1.3.1.1.2	Colonic Constipation (deleted in 1998)
1.3.1.2	Diarrhea
1.3.1.3	Bowel Incontinence
1.3.1.4	Risk for Constipation
1.3.2	Altered Urinary Elimination
1.3.2.1.1	Stress Incontinence
1.3.2.1.2	Reflex Urinary Incontinence
1.3.2.1.3	Urge Incontinence
1.3.2.1.4	Functional Urinary Incontinence
1.3.2.1.5	Total Incontinence
1.3.2.1.6	Risk for Urinary Urge Incontinence
1.3.2.2	Urinary Retention
1.4.1.1	Altered Tissue Perfusion (Specify type: Renal, Cerebral, Cardiopulmonary, Gastrointestinal, Peripheral)
1.4.1.2	Risk for Fluid Volume Imbalance

continues

Exhibit 5–3 continued

1.4.1.2.1	Fluid Volume Excess
1.4.1.2.2.1	Fluid Volume Deficit
1.4.1.2.2.2	Risk for Fluid Volume Deficit
1.4.2.1	Decreased Cardiac Output
1.5.1.1	Impaired Gas Exchange
1.5.1.2	Ineffective Airway Clearance
1.5.1.3	Ineffective Breathing Pattern
1.5.1.3.1	Inability to Sustain Spontaneous Ventilation
1.5.1.3.2	Dysfunctional Ventilatory Weaning Response
1.6.1	Risk for Injury
1.6.1.1	Risk for Suffocation
1.6.1.2	Risk for Poisoning
1.6.1.3	Risk for Trauma
1.6.1.4	Risk for Aspiration
1.6.1.5	Risk for Disuse Syndrome
1.6.1.6	Latex Allergy Response
1.6.1.7	Risk for Latex Allergy Response
1.6.2	Altered Protection
1.6.2.1	Impaired Tissue Integrity
1.6.2.1.1	Altered Oral Mucous Membrane
1.6.2.1.2.1	Impaired Skin Integrity
1.6.2.1.2.2	Risk for Impaired Skin Integrity
1.6.2.1.3	Altered Dentition
1.7.1	Decreased Adaptive Capacity: Intracranial
1.8	Energy Field Disturbance
Pattern 2: Communicating	
2.1.1.1	Impaired Verbal Communication
Pattern 3: Relating	
3.1.1	Impaired Social Interaction
3.1.2	Social Isolation
3.1.3	Risk for Loneliness
3.2.1	Altered Role Performance
3.2.1.1.1	Altered Parenting
3.2.1.1.2	Risk for Altered Parenting
3.2.1.1.2.1	Risk for Altered Parent/Infant/Child Attachment
3.2.1.2.1	Sexual Dysfunction
3.2.2	Altered Family Processes
3.2.2.1	Caregiver Role Strain
3.2.2.2	Risk for Caregiver Role Strain
3.2.2.3.1	Altered Family Process: Alcoholism
3.2.3.1	Parental Role Conflict
3.3	Altered Sexuality Patterns
Pattern 4: Valuing	
4.1.1	Spiritual Distress (Distress of the Human Spirit)
4.1.2	Risk for Spiritual Distress
4.2	Potential for Enhanced Spiritual Well-Being

continues

Exhibit 5–3 continued

Pattern 5: Choosing

5.1.1.1	Ineffective Individual Coping
5.1.1.1.1	Impaired Adjustment
5.1.1.1.2	Defensive Coping
5.1.1.1.3	Ineffective Denial
5.1.2.1.1	Ineffective Family Coping: Disabling
5.1.2.1.2	Ineffective Family Coping: Compromised
5.1.2.2	Family Coping: Potential for Growth
5.1.3.1	Potential for Enhanced Community Coping
5.1.3.2	Ineffective Community Coping
5.2.1	Ineffective Management of Therapeutic Regimen: Individuals
5.2.1.1	Noncompliance (specify)
5.2.2	Ineffective Management of Therapeutic Regimen: Families
5.2.3	Ineffective Management of Therapeutic Regimen: Community
5.2.4	Effective Management of Therapeutic Regimen: Individual
5.3.1.1	Decisional Conflict (specify)
5.4	Health-Seeking Behaviors (specify)

Pattern 6: Moving

6.1.1.1	Impaired Physical Mobility
6.1.1.1.1	Risk for Peripheral Neurovascular Dysfunction
6.1.1.1.2	Risk for Perioperative Positioning Injury
6.1.1.1.3	Impaired Walking
6.1.1.1.4	Impaired Wheelchair Mobility
6.1.1.1.5	Impaired Transfer Ability
6.1.1.1.6	Impaired Bed Mobility
6.1.1.2	Activity Intolerance
6.1.1.2.1	Fatigue
6.1.1.3	Risk for Activity Intolerance
6.2.1	Sleep Pattern Disturbance
6.2.1.1	Sleep Deprivation
6.3.1.1	Diversional Activity Deficit
6.4.1.1	Impaired Home Maintenance Management
6.4.2	Altered Health Maintenance
6.4.2.1	Delayed Surgical Recovery
6.4.2.2	Adult Failure To Thrive
6.5.1	Feeding Self-Care Deficit
6.5.1.1	Impaired Swallowing
6.5.1.2	Ineffective Breastfeeding
6.5.1.2.1	Interrupted Breastfeeding
6.5.1.3	Effective Breastfeeding
6.5.1.4	Ineffective Infant Feeding Pattern
6.5.2	Bathing/Hygiene Self-Care Deficit
6.5.3	Dressing/Grooming Self-Care Deficit
6.5.4	Toileting Self-Care Deficit
6.6	Altered Growth and Development

continues

Exhibit 5–3 continued

6.6.1	Risk for Altered Development
6.6.2	Risk for Altered Growth
6.7	Relocation Stress Syndrome
6.8.1	Risk for Disorganized Infant Behavior
6.8.2	Disorganized Infant Behavior
6.8.3	Potential for Enhanced Organized Infant Behavior

Pattern 7: Perceiving

7.1.1	Body Image Disturbance
7.1.2	Self-Esteem Disturbance
7.1.2.1	Chronic Low Self-Esteem
7.1.2.2	Situational Low Self-Esteem
7.1.3	Personal Identity Disturbance
7.2	Sensory/Perceptual Alterations (Specify: Visual, Auditory, Kinesthetic, Gustatory, Tactile, Olfactory)
7.2.1.1	Unilateral Neglect
7.3.1	Hopelessness
7.3.2	Powerlessness

Pattern 8: Knowing

8.1.1	Knowledge Deficit (Specify)
8.2.1	Impaired Environmental Interpretation Syndrome
8.2.2	Acute Confusion
8.2.3	Chronic Confusion
8.3	Altered Thought Processes
8.3.1	Impaired Memory

Pattern 9: Feeling

9.1.1	Pain
9.1.1.1	Chronic Pain
9.1.2	Nausea
9.2.1.1	Dysfunctional Grieving
9.2.1.2	Anticipatory Grieving
9.2.1.3	Chronic Sorrow
9.2.2	Risk for Violence: Directed at Others
9.2.2.1	Risk for Self-Mutilation
9.2.2.2	Risk for Violence: Self-Directed
9.2.3	Post-Trauma Response
9.2.3.1	Rape-Trauma Syndrome
9.2.3.1.1	Rape-Trauma Syndrome: Compound Reaction
9.2.3.1.2	Rape-Trauma Syndrome: Silent Reaction
9.2.4	Risk for Post-Trauma Syndrome
9.3.1	Anxiety
9.3.1.1	Death Anxiety
9.3.2	Fear

Source: Reprinted with permission from North American Nursing Diagnosis Association (1999). *NANDA Nursing Diagnoses: Definitions and Classification 1999–2000,* Philadelphia: NANDA.

Risk diagnoses are those that describe "human responses to health conditions and life processes that may develop in a vulnerable individual, family, or community."[9] Risk diagnoses are written together with risk factors that contribute to the increased vulnerability (e.g., risk for altered nutrition: less than body requirements related to nausea, vomiting, fatigue, and activity intolerance because of chemotherapy).[2]

Wellness diagnoses describe "human responses to levels of wellness in an individual, family, or community that have a potential for enhancement to a higher state"[9] (e.g., potential for enhanced adjustment to illness).[2] Wellness diagnoses have enlarged the diagnostic labeling process from an illness-centered perspective to one that integrates wellness and the preventive and curative nursing roles.[1]

Kelley, Frisch, and Avant have conceptualized the links between actual, risk, and wellness diagnoses in their trifocal model of nursing diagnoses.[14] The trifocal model, which demonstrates the movement toward health and wellness through a pyramid, expands current thinking of nursing diagnoses to permit use of the current list of NANDA's diagnostic labels in prevention and wellness. Within this trifocal model (Figure 5–1) there are three levels of nursing practice: care of an identified nursing problem (i.e., the base of the pyramid), care to prevent a problem when the nurse assesses that the client is at risk (i.e., the middle section of the pyramid), and care directed toward enhancing the client's current level of harmony, balance, and wellness (i.e., the top of the pyramid). The trifocal model permits the nurse to perceive and depict a multidimensional portrait of the client, who demonstrates balance and harmony in the midst of experiencing actual or potential illness.[2] The exciting part of this model is that any of NANDA's current diagnostic labels can be used at each of the three levels. Using the model and the terms *problem, risk for . . .* and *opportunity to enhance* provides nurses with a framework to use NANDA's nursing diagnoses during all levels of nurse-client encounters.[14] In addition, the model provides a visual tool that can serve as a communication and teaching device to use with clients in validating patterns/problems/needs and life processes and creating a collaborative plan of care.

The diagnostic process involves clinical reasoning that incorporates reflective concurrent, creative, and critical thinking to understand the client's story and organize nursing actions to achieve desired client outcomes.[15] Listening to the client's story, connecting with their experience, and uncovering the facts and the meaning surrounding their situation are key elements in clinical reasoning. Such activities permit the nurse to create a mental model, or a frame, that helps to understand the client's world, distinguish between central and peripheral problems, identify the major concerns, and take action.[15] The frame then influences and guides perception and behavior. Linking facts and cues in a logical way and retrieving specific patterns of knowing from past experiences also are a part of clinical reasoning.[15]

During the assessment, nurses determine what data are significant and what data are not. As the assessment process is begun, information is immediately clustered and processed. As the assessment continues, the data are continuously categorized, synthesized, analyzed, evaluated, and finally interpreted so that conclusions can be drawn for the purposes of diagnostic labeling.[16] Before making a specific nursing diagnosis, however, the nurse first assesses the defining characteristics (observable cues and inferences) that cluster together as manifestations of the problem. In addition to the partial list of published defining characteristics that assist nurses in verifying a particular nursing diagnosis, nurses must also use their knowledge, education, experience, clinical reasoning skills, and intuition to confirm the existence of the pattern/problem/need and life processes identified.[2]

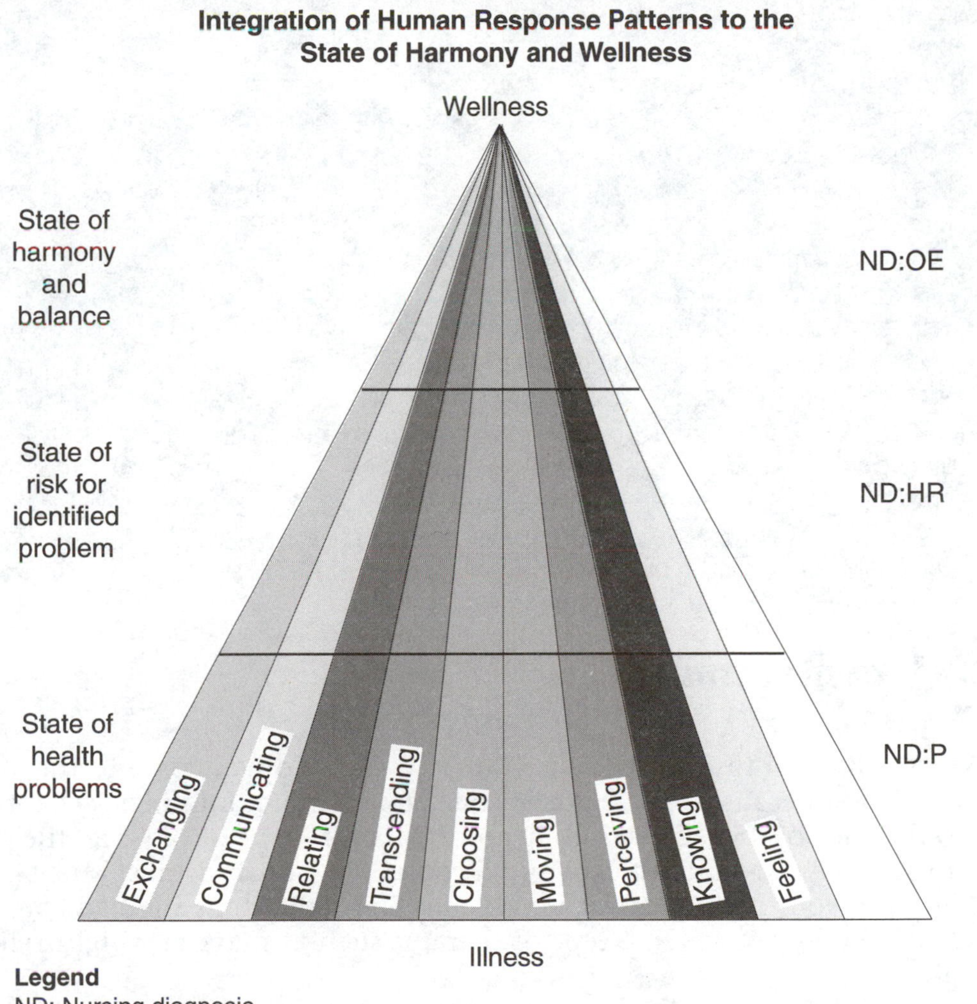

Figure 5–1 Trifocal Model of Nursing Diagnosis. *Source:* Reprinted with permission from J. Kelley, N. Frisch, and K. Avant, A Trifocal Model of Nursing Diagnosis: Wellness Revisited, *Nursing Diagnosis*, Vol. 6, pp. 123–128, © 1995, North American Nursing Diagnosis Association.

Holistic nurses understand that nursing diagnoses provide the language for describing a client's health pattern manifestations. Nursing diagnoses provide a descriptive tool for articulating human responses identified in the nurse-client relationship, but they are not intended to be constrictive diagnostic labels that might limit or stereotype care.[2] The client's, not the nurse's, values, intuitive perceptions, and meaning attached to the experience are the foundation for holistic nursing decisions and diagnostic labeling. In contrast to the biomedical tradition in which the physician often diagnoses patient problems in isolation, holistic nurses realize that they alone cannot determine what is wrong with clients and what is best for them. Thus, whenever possible, the nurse shares with the client and other health team members the patterns and strengths recognized from the assessment and the client, in turn, validates both the existence and meaning of these identified response patterns.

It is critical that clients also take part in prioritizing the patterns/problems/needs, because when nurses plan care for a problem that does not have major relevance to the client's perceived concerns, efforts to achieve desired outcomes are often futile. Likewise, clients whose primary concerns are neglected or postponed often do not progress as expected.[3] The list of nursing diagnoses, therefore, should be prioritized based on the client's most immediate perceived patterns/problems/needs gathered from the client's story and validated by the client's perception.

Patterns/problems/needs that have been identified, validated, and prioritized with the client form the basis of the remaining steps of the holistic caring process. They must be documented in the client's record for the purposes of planning care and communicating the client's status to all involved members of the health care team.

CASE STUDIES

1 Nurse Elizabeth introduced herself to Mrs. G., who had come to the Wellness Center because of an acute episode of pain in her lower back that traveled to the back of the leg and into her foot. Mrs. G., 49 years old, said the pain began three days ago after picking up a cooler full of soft drinks. Mrs. G. denied any previous history of back problems. She stated that she had come to the Center hoping that some type of therapy, such as massage, might relieve the pain.

During Mrs. G.'s health assessment, Elizabeth learned that Mrs. G.'s husband, who had been at home convalescing for nine weeks from a broken leg, had recently undergone a second surgery because of complications. In addition, her 15-year-old daughter was going through a rebellious stage, skipping school, sneaking out late at night, and dating the "boyfriend from hell." Moreover, the security of her current job as a publisher and her financial future were uncertain because her publishing house had just been merged with a larger company.

Elizabeth shared the findings of her assessment with Mrs. G. "Mrs. G., it is my understanding that you came here seeking some relief from your back and leg pain. I would like to recommend that you be assessed by our licensed acupuncturist here at the Center. There is research evidence that acupuncture can be a useful treatment in the management of problems such as yours.[17] The acupuncturist will determine whether acupuncture treatments might help you and will discuss the type of sessions and possible length of the treatment." Elizabeth also shared information about simple stretching exercises and over-the-counter analgesics that might be beneficial. She continued by exploring other insights she had about Mrs. G.'s situation. "Mrs. G., it also is clear that you are a caring, organized, and responsible wife and mother. From what you have told me, however, it sounds like it has been difficult to juggle all of your roles in the past three months with your daughter and sick husband. My guess is that you have had to assume the majority of responsibilities at home. I also perceive that you are very adept in your many roles but because of the stressors you've recently experienced, I sense that perhaps you are somewhat overwhelmed by it all." Mrs. G. admitted to feeling out of control lately and said, "One might go so far as to guess that all this stress contributed to my current back and leg problems." Elizabeth nodded, acknowledging Mrs. G.'s insight into the current situation. They agreed that acute stress related to personal and job-associated factors was a problem that warranted management. Mrs. G. decided to return to the clinic for an acupuncture evaluation and follow-up with Elizabeth to work on stress management and relaxation strategies.

Elizabeth is practicing the Standards that support identification of the client's patterns/problems/needs. She validates the existence and priority of the client's most pressing concern (i.e., pain), refers the client to the appropriate holistic practitioner for a therapy that is validated by research,[17] and offers advice for supportive measures such as stretching and analgesics. Thus Elizabeth begins where the client is in developing outcomes and a plan of care. Because of a thorough assessment of the client's nine human response patterns, however, Elizabeth is able to identify a more complex response pattern manifested by Mrs. G.'s strengths and coping skills as well as her responses to family, occupational, and financial stressors. After she shares this insight with the client, Mrs. G. is able to access her inner wisdom to recognize the association between her acute situation and the events of the past several months. In doing so, the client validates the meaning associated with her condition and recognizes the need to manage her stress. Elizabeth has provided the client with the opportunity to enhance her movement toward health and well-being.

2 Nurse Ashley admitted Mr. J., 61 years old, to the coronary care unit with the chief complaint of chest pain without radiation. During Ashley's assessment, she discovered that the patient has had no prior history of chest pain or heart disease. He stated, however, that he has had chills, fatigue, headache, and a poor appetite, all of which began about 10 days ago. Mr. J. revealed that as a child he had rheumatic fever and subsequently developed a murmur of mitral regurgitation. By astute interviewing skills, Ashley learned that one month ago the patient had an abscessed tooth extracted but had not received antimicrobial prophylaxis before or after the procedure. Ashley also noted during the interview that the patient was highly anxious, as demonstrated by constant talking, darting eye movements, startle reflex to normal sounds, and continuous nonpurposeful foot activity. In addition, his temporal and jaw muscles were tensed.

Upon physical examination the patient's temperature was 101.4° F orally, apical pulse 110 beats per minute, respirations 16/minute, and blood pressure 124/86 mmHg. The patient's oral hygiene was poor. Bilateral conjunctival petechiae were noted. Heart sounds were normal but a grade 3/6 holosystolic heart murmur was heard at the lower left sternal border with radiation to the left axilla. Ashley also noticed splinter hemorrhages on the distal third of the nails on the middle finger of both hands. The patient was in normal sinus rhythm with normal ECG findings. Following the consultation from the cardiologist, the patient was placed on bed rest, a 2-gm sodium diet, and cardiac monitoring. Laboratory studies were ordered, including aerobic and anaerobic blood cultures.

Ashley recorded her findings on the admission assessment form, clustered, synthesized, evaluated, and interpreted the data, and wrote the following diagnoses on the patterns/problems/needs list of the patient's medical record:

- Infection (possible cardiac valve infection—awaiting further data)
- Knowledge deficit related to acute illness and the need for prophylactic antibiotics to prevent cardiac valve infection
- Anxiety related to acute illness

Ashley's thorough assessment of Mr. J.'s condition reveals several discerning signs and symptoms that suggest the patient might be suffering from infective endocarditis. Regardless of which type of assessment framework Ashley might have used to organize and record her data, however, it is apparent that most of her information is related to the medical disease with little emphasis on understanding the patient's story. Had Ashley used the nine human response patterns as her organizing framework for data collection, for example, she would have discovered major holes in her assessment. She did not assess the human response patterns of relating (e.g., the patient's role and socialization status), valuing (e.g., religious, spiritual, and cultural concerns), knowing (e.g., the patient's perception of this illness, and possible treatment), feeling (e.g., validating Mr. J.'s current emotional integrity), perceiving (e.g., self-concept and meaningfulness), and choosing (e.g., coping, participation in health care).

Ashley's skillful assessment and diagnoses, which would fulfill the assessment requirements in most critical care units, reveals perceptive information pertinent to understanding and treating the patient's medical illness. She does not meet the Standards of Practice in identifying the patient's patterns/problems/needs, however, because she does not identify the patient's inherent strengths and potential for enhanced growth and development. She assumes she knows what is wrong and how things should be treated. Moreover, Ashley makes no attempt to validate the meaning of the illness with the patient or to validate with him the existence or priority of the other patterns/problems/needs identified.

5.3 Outcomes

■■ Each person's actual and potential patterns/problems/needs have appropriate outcomes specified. ■■

Desired client outcomes are identified for each actual, risk, or wellness diagnosis. Outcomes become the road map for clinical decision making and the plan of care. There are two Standards of Practice that demonstrate the Core Value related to identifying outcomes, as described and illustrated below.

Standard of Practice 5.3.1

Holistic nurses honor the person in all phases of her/his healing process regardless of expectations or outcomes.

Standard of Practice 5.3.2

Holistic nurses identify and partner with the person to specify measurable outcomes and realistic goals.

These Standards emphasize the Core Value that holistic nurses place on partnering and collaborating with the client to identify measurable outcomes for each nursing diagnosis that are relevant and consistent with the client's condition, needs, and desires. During this phase of the holistic caring process, the outcomes are collaboratively decided based on the client's expectations and his or her level of motivation and commitment to move toward healing endpoints. Furthermore, the Standards dictate that regardless of personal beliefs and assumptions, holistic nurses honor and respect the client's expectations and goals in achieving end results.

Table 5–3 illustrates the nursing knowledge and skills required for a nurse to meet Standards 5.3.1 and 5.3.2.

Table 5–3 Nursing Knowledge and Skills in Identifying Outcomes

Standard of Practice 5.3.1	*Key Concepts*	*Requisite Knowledge*	*Requisite Skills*
Holistic nurses honor the person in all phases of her/his healing process regardless of expectations or outcomes.	Honoring the client. Phases of healing process. Honoring client's expectations and outcomes.	Knowledge of bio-psycho-social-spiritual healing process. Honoring, respecting, and valuing client's expectations and goals for healing.	Skills in "knowing" clients to understand their expectations and goals. Experience in communicating respect for client's expectations and goals during nurse-client encounters.

continues

Table 5–3 continued

Standard of Practice 5.3.2	*Key Concepts*	*Requisite Knowledge*	*Requisite Skills*
Holistic nurses identify and partner with the person to specify measurable outcomes and realistic goals.	Partnering with client. Identifying measurable outcomes. Identifying realistic goals.	Knowledge of client outcome statements. Knowledge of outcome indicators that defined desired end result. Knowledge of tools to measure and track the trajectory of client outcomes.	Ability to compare client's current status to proposed desired outcomes. Skills in partnering with client in identifying desired outcomes. Proficiency in identifying outcome indicators and using tools to measure outcomes. Documentation of nurse-client collaborated outcomes.

Nursing Activities

For each nursing diagnosis identified, specific client outcomes are developed that reasonably can be expected to occur as a result of holistic nursing care. When outcomes are associated with care, the "process" is the care delivered (i.e., assessment, diagnosis, identification of outcomes, plan, intervention, and evaluation) and the outcome is the desired or end result of that process.[18] Outcomes are then evaluated to determine which interventions have been successful in achieving the outcome, which ones need modification, and which ones need improvement. Accreditation organizations, such as the Joint Commission on Accreditation of Healthcare Organizations, have redesigned their reviews to focus more on outcomes and less on the process used to achieve the outcomes.

Following identification of a problem, the nurse compares the client's current status to a proposed desired outcome. Such a comparison provides an image of where the client currently is and where it is desired that he or she be. Clinical decisions regarding choices of interventions are then made to bridge the gap between where the client is and what must be done to move the client to the desired state of healing.[15]

Because individuals are viewed as active participants in their health and wellness, they share responsibility and accountability for reaching their optimal outcomes.[19] If outcomes are to be achieved, clients must be empowered to achieve them, motivated to establish healthy patterns of behavior, and committed to move toward the desired changes.[2] Moreover, outcomes must be relevant to each person's purpose in seeking care. It is the client's, not the nurse's, values, expectations, and meaning attached to what is to be accomplished in the healing process that are the foundation for developing client outcomes.

Thus, outcomes are discussed and collaborated on with the client and family so that nurse and client will have a shared objective for their work together.[1] Nurses partner with the client to identify outcomes that signify the maximum level of wellness that is reasonably attainable for the client and compatible with what the client hopes to achieve based on the client's condition and perceptions.[20] In contrast, when nurses independently assume the responsibility for identifying desired outcomes that are not consistent with the client's needs (as is often the case), outcomes frequently are not achieved. Although family and other health care members may participate in developing outcomes, outcomes are direct statements of the nurse-client-identified end results to be achieved.[2]

Many kinds of client outcomes have been suggested in health care, including those related to physiologic and psychologic status, functional measures, behavior, knowledge, control of signs and symptoms, quality of life, home functioning, family strain, goal attainment, use of services, safety, problem resolution, and caring.[19,21] The six major quality indicators linking nursing care with patient outcomes that have been identified by the ANA include patient and family satisfaction, rate of adverse incidents (e.g., medication errors, patient falls), complications (e.g., pressure ulcers, hospital-acquired infections), the patient's adherence to the discharge plan, mortality rate, and the patient's length of hospital stay.[22]

Outcomes, which are usually quantifiable and reproducible, are evaluated by the criteria or outcome indicators that define the desired condition.[15,18] Outcome indicators (e.g., reduced anxiety) are developed in a way that they can be measured by tools or scales (e.g., using the visual analog scale for anxiety).[23] Knowing what to measure, however, is the challenge. Nurses can develop outcome indicators that delineate several kinds of end results, such as the circumstances that should or should not occur in a client's status; the level at which some change should occur; the client's verbalization about what he or she knows, understands, perceives, or feels about a situation; or specific client states, behaviors, signs and symptoms, or perceptions that are expected to occur as a result of an intervention.[2]

Outcome indicators are evaluated by specific tools that determine whether the outcome has been achieved. Such tools can include physiologic parameters and tests, observations, personal statements, clinical pathways, variance tracking methods, clinical complication worksheets or reports, psycho-social-spiritual scales (e.g., for anxiety, coping, quality of life), functional status scales, satisfaction surveys, process improvement monitors (i.e., quality improvement methods), administrative databases or cost accounting systems, and data collection forms from research protocols.[19]

The Nursing Outcomes Classification (NOC), developed at the University of Iowa College of Nursing, has been highly successful in standardizing patient outcomes for all clinical settings in which nurses practice. This group has defined an outcome as a "variable concept representing a patient or family-caregiver state, behavior, or perception that is measurable along a continuum and responsive to nursing interventions" (also called nurse-sensitive outcomes).[24]

NOC addresses outcomes (rather than goals) for clients with specific medical and nursing diagnoses as well as specifying outcomes for prevention, health maintenance, and health promotion. The current NOC contains over 200 outcomes and is being continually expanded, validated, and evaluated.[25] The outcomes are organized into six domains: (1) functional health, (2) physiologic health, (3) psychosocial health, (4) health knowledge and behavior, (5) perceived health, and (6) family health.

Each of the 200 outcomes has a set of indicators used to assist the nurse in evaluating the client's outcome status. In addition, each outcome includes measurement scales to rate the client's outcome status, which can be assessed at various points in time so that trends in the client's progress in response to nursing interventions can be evaluated, mapped, and documented. By using these measurement scales, holistic nurses can identify positive or negative changes or no change in the client's status by evaluating the outcomes at several different points in time during the holistic caring process.[25]

For example, health care knowledge is an important client outcome that is sensitive to nursing intervention. It is uncommonly documented by other health care disciplines and often is not visible in interdisciplinary outcome measures.[25] Holistic nurses play a major role in educating clients so that they can understand and make informed decisions about health care options and healthy lifestyle behaviors. As a result of the education, it is hoped that the client's knowledge and understanding will be increased. It is postulated that such increased understanding will provide the client with more self-confidence about healthy choices, which in turn will positively change the client's self-care behavior to improve his or her health and functional status. Client education thus is often measured at different points in time to determine whether the client has indeed achieved a better level of understanding. In turn, additional measurement is often necessary to determine whether the patient actually has changed his or her behavior and whether such changes have resulted in improved health and wellness.[18]

Holistic nurses can communicate and document their contribution to the healing, health, and well-being of individuals by using the language of standardized outcomes in practice. In addition, using standardized nurse-sensitive patient outcomes makes the effects of nursing care more visible, increases nursing's accountability in all phases of client healing and health, and specifically demonstrates the effects of nursing care on clients. Likewise, holistic nurses can use standardized client outcomes to create databases, document the healing effects of care, and facilitate research efforts (e.g., by comparing the effects of various nursing interventions in achieving successful outcomes).[25] Because of the current value placed on outcomes by both professional and consumer groups, outcomes also have the potential to be translated into powerful health care decisions that foster holistic healing practices.

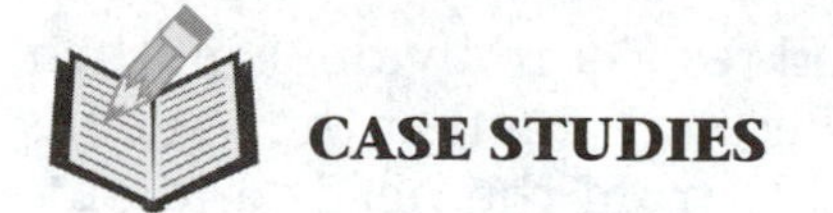

CASE STUDIES

1 Nurse Dezra was working on the Trauma Service when Lonny, a 13-year-old boy, was brought into the emergency department (ED) following a motor vehicle collision in which the patient was ejected from the back seat of his car. His mother and father, who also were in the car, had minimal injuries and were at Lonny's side rendering aid when the Emergency Medical Services arrived at the scene. It was determined that Lonny had sustained severe head, chest, and abdominal trauma. During his transport to the hospital, he went into full cardiopulmonary arrest. CPR was initiated during transport and continued on admission to the ED.

Dezra was notified that Lonny's mother and father had arrived at the ED and were asking to see their son. Dezra went to the family waiting room to update the parents on the seriousness of Lonny's condition and describe the resuscitation that was taking place. Lonny's parents told Dezra that they wanted to see their son. With compassion, Dezra explained that families are not allowed in the trauma room when patients are undergoing CPR but promised to check on their son's current status and see what she could do. Upon returning to the trauma room, Dezra found the team involved in continued resuscitative efforts.

Sensing that the patient's outcome would not be favorable, Dezra told the attending trauma surgeon that Lonny's parents were insistent about seeing their son. She explained that they had been with him during the accident but had not seen him since transport. She related that after the parents had been sufficiently briefed about their son's current condition and the activities in the room, they were even more determined to see Lonny. She conveyed to the surgeon that it was her opinion, after assessing the stability of the parents' emotional state, that bedside visitation was an appropriate intervention for these parents in meeting their immediate needs. She told the surgeon she would prepare the family for the visit, escort them to the bedside and stay with them during a brief visit, and assume the responsibility for their appropriate behavior. Reluctantly, the surgeon agreed to the visitation.

Dezra returned to the family and informed them about Lonny's deteriorating condition, and then briefly painted a picture of what they could expect to see and hear at the bedside. The family remained adamant that they needed to see and talk to him, if possible. Dezra reassured them that the sense of hearing is often the last to go and that it was possible that Lonny would hear their voices. She escorted the family to their son's bedside, cleared a place for them to stand at the head of the bed, touched Lonny's forehead, and told him that his parents were there. Without any hesitation, the parents knew what to do. They told Lonny to be strong and to hold on. They told him how much they loved him. Lonny's father apologized for the argument they had just before the accident. They touched their son and kissed his forehead. They prayed. Dezra then escorted the parents back to the family room and supported them until they received word a few minutes later that Lonny had died. Several weeks after Lonny's death, Dezra received a letter from his parents thanking her for making it possible to share the precious gift of their son's last living minutes.

Dezra is practicing the Standards that honor and respect individuals in their healing journey regardless of their expectations. Recognizing that the patient's death is imminent, the focus of Dezra's care shifts from the needs and outcomes of the patient to those of the family. Lonny's parents plainly state their needs and goals. Dezra listens to their story and recognizes that bedside visitation could meet their need for seeing, hearing about, and understanding Lonny's critical condition as well as for furnishing connectedness and closure with him. Dezra senses that bringing Lonny's parents to their son's bedside is without question the right thing to do. She both honors and respects their wishes and therefore considers the family presence option despite universal institutional rules that prohibit such practice. Moreover, in assessing the parents' reactions and behaviors during her encounters with them, Dezra makes the clinical judgment that the parents likely would be emotionally able to cope with the experience. Having made this decision, her plan of action becomes clear.

As the family advocate, she then intervenes on their behalf by talking to the trauma surgeon about their bedside visitation and offering a compelling and reasonable plan to make it happen. In addition to playing the role of family advocate and bedside facilitator, Dezra also becomes a coach by modeling how to talk to and touch Lonny, demonstrating how to *be with* the patient in a strange and frightening environment to transform their role from passive observers to active participants. She is aware that even in the midst of this devastating crisis, healing is possible for this family. In offering the gift of presence, Dezra bestows a sense of groundedness, a centering influence, and a transcendent quality that helps the family rise above the chaos to gain understanding, perspective, and meaning.[26]

2 Nurse Dorrie had never taken care of Mrs. L. until her cardiac arrest. The resuscitation was successful and the patient survived. The next day during morning report, Dorrie asked to be assigned to Mrs. L. As she entered the patient's room, she introduced herself, explained she had been part of the team taking care of her yesterday, and told Mrs. L. that she was happy she was doing so well. Mrs. L. smiled and said, "I know all of that. But did you know that it is because of you that I am here?" Dorrie said she didn't understand. Mrs. L. went on to explain that while they were doing CPR on her, she saw everything that was going on. She described the people in the room and the events of the experience. She related that she was ready to leave the room when she felt a tap on her shoulder, saw Dorrie at her bedside, and knew she had to return. Dorrie explained to Mrs. L. that it was really the successful efforts of the medical team that brought Mrs. L. back. She suggested to Mrs. L. that she talk to a specialist about this experience and arranged for the psychosocial clinical nurse specialist to visit with Mrs. L. that afternoon.

Dorrie's request to care for Mrs. L. and her sincere joy in seeing her doing so well the day after the cardiac arrest demonstrated a high level of caring and responsiveness to the patient. Dorrie did not comply with Standards 5.3.1 and 5.3.2, however, because she made the clinical decision that she had nothing to offer and was incapable of meeting the client's immediate needs. She made the psychosocial referral to assist Mrs. L. in processing her near-death experience, believing that someone else had the answers. Because she felt ill prepared to deal with such issues, she did not recognize that her caring presence was perhaps the most powerful resource at the moment for this client. It was clear that Mrs. L. credited Dorrie with her return to life and likely had a need to process this experience with her. The outcome of such a caring exchange might have provided Mrs. L. with the insight to uncover the meaning and purpose surrounding this powerful event. Had Dorrie accepted the opportunity to become engaged with Mrs. L. in a healing encounter, she might have discovered that there were no right answers in helping Mrs. L. and that only her presence and caring were necessary to release the patient's inherent healing response.

5.4 Therapeutic Care Plan

■■ ***Each person engages with the holistic nurse to mutually create an appropriate plan of care that focuses on health promotion, recovery, restoration, or peaceful dying so that the person is as independent as possible.*** ■■

Based on the client outcomes identified, care is planned to achieve the desired end results for health promotion, recovery from illness, restoration of health, or peaceful dying. In collaboration with the client, the plan is established to repattern behaviors, achieve a healthier state, and foster client independence. Six Standards of Practice demonstrate the Core Value of planning appropriate client care, as described and illustrated below.

Standard of Practice 5.4.1

Holistic nurses partner with the person in a mutual decision process to create a health care plan for each pattern/problem/need or opportunity to enhance health and well-being.

Standard of Practice 5.4.2

Holistic nurses help a person identify areas for education to make decisions about life choices in a conscious, informed manner that empowers the person to maintain her/his uniqueness and independence.

Standard of Practice 5.4.3

Holistic nurses offer self-assessment tools, word associations, storytelling, dreams, journals as appropriate.

Standard of Practice 5.4.4

Holistic nurses use skills of cultural competence and communicate acceptance of the person's values, beliefs, culture, religion, and socioeconomic background.

Standard of Practice 5.4.5

Holistic nurses assist the person in recognizing at-risk patterns/problems/needs for potential or existing health situations (e.g., personal habits, personal and family health history, age-related risk factors), and also assist in recognizing opportunities to enhance well-being.

Standard of Practice 5.4.6

Holistic nurses engage the person in problem-solving dialogue in relation to living with changes secondary to illness and treatment.

These Standards underscore the value that holistic nurses place on partnering and collaborating with the client to create a plan of care that empowers individuals to maintain their uniqueness and independence. The need to educate clients to enable them to make informed decisions about lifestyle changes and healthy behaviors and provide opportunities for clients to enhance their health and well-being is emphasized. The client outcomes direct the plan of care. To achieve successful client outcomes, each intervention is chosen based on its potential clinical effectiveness as well as its acceptability to the client in terms of the client's values, beliefs, culture, religion, and socioeconomic background. These Standards also outline the nurse's role as a client facilitator and advocate in customizing the plan of care to achieve desired, future-state outcomes.

Table 5–4 illustrates the nursing knowledge and skills required for a nurse to meet Standards 5.4.1, 5.4.2, 5.4.3, 5.4.4, 5.4.5, and 5.4.6.

Table 5–4 Nursing Knowledge and Skills in Planning Care

Standard of Practice 5.4.1	*Key Concepts*	*Requisite Knowledge*	*Requisite Skills*
Holistic nurses partner with the person in a mutual decision process to create a health care plan for each pattern/problem/need or opportunity to enhance health and well-being.	Partner with client. Mutual decision process. Health care plan for each pattern/problem/need. Opportunity to enhance health and well-being.	Knowledge of health care planning. Understanding strategies to enhance health and well-being.	Experience in planning care to achieve outcomes. Skills in collaborating with client to create plan of care.

continues

Table 5–4 continued

Standard of Practice 5.4.1	*Key Concepts*	*Requisite Knowledge*	*Requisite Skills*
		Knowing clients and their story, perceptions, and goals.	Ability to provide opportunities to support and enhance client in movement toward health and well-being. Documentation of the client-nurse plan of care.

Standard of Practice 5.4.2	*Key Concepts*	*Requisite Knowledge*	*Requisite Skills*
Holistic nurses help a person identify areas for education to make decisions about life choices in a conscious, informed manner that empowers the person to maintain her/his uniqueness and independence.	Client education. Conscious, informed decisions about life choices. Client empowerment. Maintenance of client's uniqueness and independence.	Principles of client education. Knowledge of life choice options. Principles of informed decision making.	Client guidance to identify educational needs. Client education skills. Empowering clients with knowledge to choose healthy behaviors. Valuing the client's uniqueness and need for independence. Communication skills that reflect respect for client as a unique and independent being.

Standard of Practice 5.4.3	*Key Concepts*	*Requisite Knowledge*	*Requisite Skills*
Holistic nurses offer self-assessment tools, word associations, storytelling, dreams, journals as appropriate.	Offering and guiding clients in using self-assessments, word associations, storytelling, dreams, and journals.	Knowledge of and understanding in using self-assessments, word associations, storytelling, dreams, and journals with clients.	Skills in offering client self-assessments, word associations, storytelling, dreams, and journals in understanding the client's story and meaning associated with health and wellness.

continues

Table 5–4 continued

Standard of Practice 5.4.3	*Key Concepts*	*Requisite Knowledge*	*Requisite Skills*
			Reflection skills communicating insights gained from self-assessments.

Standard of Practice 5.4.4	*Key Concepts*	*Requisite Knowledge*	*Requisite Skills*
Holistic nurses use skills of cultural competence and communicate acceptance of the person's values, beliefs, culture, religion, and socioeconomic background.	Use skills of cultural competence. Communicate acceptance. Client's values, beliefs, culture, religion, and socioeconomic background.	Knowledge of cultural differences and culturally competent care. Recognition of nurse's own values, beliefs, culture, religion, and socioeconomic background and how such variables influence the care provided.	Skills in providing culturally competent care (i.e., ability to respect and communicate acceptance of client's values, beliefs, culture, religion, and socioeconomic status).

Standard of Practice 5.4.5	*Key Concepts*	*Requisite Knowledge*	*Requisite Skills*
Holistic nurses assist the person in recognizing at-risk patterns/ problems/needs for potential or existing health situations (e.g., personal habits, personal and family health history, age-related risk factors), and also assist in recognizing opportunities to enhance well-being.	Assist person to recognize risk patterns/ problems/needs or existing health situations. At-risk personal habits. At-risk personal and family health history. At-risk age-related factors. Recognizing opportunities to enhance health and well-being.	Knowledge of risk factors associated with personal habits, personal and family health history, or age-related risk factors for individual clients. Knowledge of strategies that provide opportunities to enhance well-being.	Collaboration skills in helping client identify risk behaviors and personal risk profiles that could progress to actual unhealthy patterns, problems, needs. Ability to provide opportunities to enhance and support the client's movement toward health and well-being.

continues

Table 5–4 continued

Standard of Practice 5.4.6	*Key Concepts*	*Requisite Knowledge*	*Requisite Skills*
Holistic nurses engage the person in problem-solving dialogue in relation to living with changes secondary to illness and treatment.	Engage the client in problem-solving dialogue. Living with changes related to illness and treatment.	Knowledge of problem-solving methods. Understanding principles of communication. Understanding need for alterations in lifestyle related to specific illness and treatments.	Skills in therapeutic communication with the client. Problem-solving skills used during client encounters. Skills in planning care with client that is realistic for the client's condition and treatment.

Nursing Activities

For each client outcome identified, specific interventions are planned. Within the planning stage of the holistic caring process, the nurse partners with the client to explore ways that clients can repattern their behaviors to achieve a healthier state. Identified outcomes become the road map for planning care. The plan outlines which nursing interventions and actions need to be performed to help the client solve problems, move toward health, and accomplish the outcomes. The plan of care directs the implementation phase of the holistic caring process.[2]

Nursing interventions are defined as "any direct care treatment that a nurse performs on behalf of a client. The treatments include nurse-initiated treatments resulting from nursing diagnoses, physician-initiated treatments resulting from medical diagnoses, and performance of daily essential functions for the client who cannot do these."[27] Priorities for outcomes and interventions are decided by determining the urgency of the pattern/problem/need to the client's safety, life, and well-being.

In planning care, the nurse needs to consider several factors when selecting the appropriate interventions to achieve outcomes.[27,28] One of the first factors to be considered is whether the intervention will be useful and effective in achieving the desired outcomes based on the characteristics of the patterns/problems/needs (i.e., whether the intervention is aimed at the etiology, signs and symptoms, or at-risk problems).[15,28] Such clinical decisions are based on a knowledge of existing research findings that validate the clinical significance and effectiveness of the intervention as well as its associated complications or adverse effects. When such a research base does not exist, nurses must rely on their clinical experience and education in choosing from among the various intervention options. Also, the degree of nursing control and the nursing competency necessary to successfully implement the intervention should be evaluated. Moreover, the feasibility of implementing the intervention is assessed related to the priority and significance of other patterns/problems/needs and examined in terms of its associated time and cost. Thus, clinical decisions about which interventions to use are based on utility, characteristics of the problem, effectiveness, nursing competency, and feasibility.[2,27,28]

Perhaps most important, however, the acceptability of the potential intervention must be discussed with clients in terms of their priorities and goals as well as their values, beliefs, culture, religion, and socioeconomic background. In partnering with the client to develop the plan of care, it may be useful to have the client assess the integration of their human potentials, including physical ability, mental ability, emotions, relationships, choices, and spirit.[29] The results of such self-assessments combined with the insight gained from storytelling, dreams, and journaling often provide clients with wisdom about their current status and what they desire to change. Such activities facilitate dialogue between the client and the nurse to process emotions, problem-solve, and discover acceptable lifestyle changes and behaviors that are consistent with barriers that may be imposed by illness states. Interventions selected during the planning phase should have relevance to clients and provide opportunities to empower them to enhance their health and maintain their uniqueness and independence. Thus, additional factors to consider when selecting appropriate interventions include the relevance and acceptability to the client as well as the potential to enhance health and well-being.[2,27,28]

To attain optimal desired client outcomes, the plan must be developed within the context of the client's cultural background, beliefs, and values related to illness and health. Culture motivates health and illness behaviors as well as patterns of responses and movement toward recovery. As nurses partner with clients in planning care, activities to promote, maintain, or restore health must be selected within a cultural context. Knowing and accepting the client's rights to alternative strategies and modalities must be incorporated into the mutually designed plan of care. Cultural healing practices should be included unless contraindicated.[30]

The clinical decision making involved in selecting appropriate interventions is aimed at helping clients make the transition from the present state to the desired outcome state.[15] Clinical judgment guides decisions about what to observe in clients to derive meaning from the data observed and what actions need to be taken to achieve optimal end results. Customized clinical decisions depend, however, on nursing presence and *knowing the client*. The judgments nurses make about their clients' problems and desired outcome states and the decisions they make about which intervention to use embody the data gathered while being present with clients.[31] When nurses are fully engaged in the client's immediate experience, they are open to the patterns and life processes that unfold. As a result of such encounters, the nurse learns "to know" the client. Knowing the client can be defined as "understanding the patient's experiences, behaviors, feelings, and/or perceptions to select individualized interventions."[32,33]

Clinical decisions that are grounded in knowing the client allow the nurse to visualize beyond the current moment to the possibilities inherent in the situation to enhance health and well-being. Knowing the client often provides the nurse with the intuitive sense about what will work. It furnishes the details surrounding the client's patterns and responses to facilitate the selection of interventions that are consistent with the client's personhood and customized to meet his or her unique and individualized needs.[32,34] Moreover, the power elicited from knowing the client and the resultant nurse-client relationship that is formed can promote the healing process.[35]

The plan of care is documented in the client's record to communicate this information to other multidisciplinary health care team members and coordinate care. Revising the plan of care is an ongoing process based on achievement of outcomes that are measured at several different points in times.

CASE STUDIES

1 Mrs. W., age 34, met Nurse Christina for the first time during her annual wellness check. Mrs. W. related her health history in a brief life review. She described her 17-year struggle with weight cycling. Although she previously had been active in sports and exercise, the demands of her job in the past few years kept her busy and prevented her from exercising regularly. She was tearful when she told of her repeated failures to lose and maintain a healthy weight and ranked herself low when presented with a body image scale.

Christina assessed Mrs. W. and determined that she was in good physical health except for her mild obesity, inactivity, and risk for binge eating. Christina shared her assessment findings with the client, discussed the health risks involved, and explained the holistic self-care model weight management program that was offered at the clinic. Christina answered Mrs. W.'s additional questions and encouraged her to call the clinic for more information when she was ready.

Two weeks later, Mrs. W. contacted the clinic to inquire about details of the weight management program's group sessions. After attending several sessions, Mrs. W. revealed that she had become aware of how much she had been eating when she was not hungry, especially when work built up at her job. She expressed more hope that she could cut down on the quantity of her food by following the eating strategy that was offered in the program. She also expressed interest in attending the next sessions on exercise offered at the clinic, although she had not changed her activity level to date.[36]

Christina is practicing the Standards that support care planning to assist the client in repatterning behaviors to achieve a healthier state. During her client's initial visit, Christina recognizes that Mrs. W. is in the contemplation stage of change. She realizes that when clients are not ready to make lifestyle changes, nurses cannot motivate them to do so.[37] Christina takes advantage of this stage, however, and shares her assessment findings with the client, discusses the risks, and furnishes Mrs. W. with the options that are available.

Christina also communicates respect for where the client is. She refrains from planning the weight management sessions and scheduling Mrs. W. for her first appointment. Thus Christina is furnishing the client with the details necessary to raise her consciousness without imposing any demands. In doing so, she creates the opportunity in which Mrs. W. is free to change at her own pace and empowered to find her own unique, individualized healing path.

2 Case Manager Nurse Jessica was preparing for Mrs. K.'s discharge after a five-week hospital stay following a complicated knee replacement. Mrs. K., 78 years old and married for 57 years, had multiple rehabilitation needs. Jessica arranged for a home care nurse to visit Mrs. K. twice a week to assess her progress, draw blood for her lab work, and change her dressings. In addition, she scheduled a physical therapist and occupational therapist for twice-weekly home visits, along with a home health aide for daily morning visits to assist Mrs. K. with bathing and personal needs. Mrs. and Mr. K. were informed of the arrangements and discharged to home. The next morning Jessica learned that Mr. K. had fired all of the arranged health care personnel, stating that he intended to care for his wife alone but was afraid to tell the nurses at the hospital because he did not want to make them angry.

Jessica's care does not comply with the Standards that support holistic care planning because she does not partner with the patient and family to discover their personal needs and expectations following discharge. In her encounters with them, she presumes that she knows what is right for this family. Jessica assumes that Mrs. K.'s rehabilitation needs are best met by health care professionals. Based on this belief, she meticulously plans Mrs. K.'s care based on the discharge outcomes to be achieved and independently arranges for the home health referrals. She makes no attempt to know the family. Her actions demonstrate a "doing to" rather than a "being with" style of practice. She does not explore the patient's and husband's story and the meaning the discharge plan has for them. Had she done so and discovered that Mr. K. planned to care for his wife alone, despite her professional misgivings Jessica would have revised her plan and worked to prepare Mr. K. before discharge for the skills, care, and responsibilities he would have encountered in caring for his wife at home.

5.5 Implementation

■■ ***Each person's plan of holistic care is prioritized and holistic nursing interventions are implemented accordingly.*** ■■

Based on the mutually derived plan of care, interventions are prioritized and implemented to achieve desired outcomes. Interventions are carried out for the purposes of promoting health, recovering from illness, restoring health, or dying in peace. There are five Standards of Practice that demonstrate the Core Value of implementing nursing interventions, as described and illustrated below.

Standard of Practice 5.5.1

Holistic nurses implement the mutually created plan of care within the context of assisting the person toward the higher potential of health and well-being.

Standard of Practice 5.5.2

Holistic nurses support and promote the person's capacity for the highest level of participation and problem solving in the plan of care and collaborate with other health team members when appropriate.

Standard of Practice 5.5.3

Holistic nurses use holistic nursing skills in implementing care including cultural competency and all ways of knowing.

Standard of Practice 5.5.4

Holistic nurses advocate that the person's plan, choices, and unique healing journey be honored.

Standard of Practice 5.5.5

Holistic nurses provide care that is clear about and respectful of the economic parameters of practice, balancing justice with compassion.

These Standards highlight the Core Values that holistic nurses place on implementing a mutually derived plan of care to help the client achieve a higher potential of health and well-being by promoting the client's highest level of participation in their own care and honoring their goals, choices, and unique healing journey. The Standards dictate that the interventions will be implemented within the context of the client's cultural background, beliefs, and values. Moreover, the collaborative role of the nurse in problem solving and in working with other health team members in achieving client outcomes is emphasized. These Standards also underscore the need to balance economic constraints with compassionate care.

Table 5–5 illustrates the nursing knowledge and skills required for a nurse to meet Standards 5.5.1, 5.5.2, 5.5.3, 5.5.4, and 5.5.5.

Table 5–5 Nursing Knowledge and Skills in Implementing Interventions

Standard of Practice 5.5.1	*Key Concepts*	*Requisite Knowledge*	*Requisite Skills*
Holistic nurses implement the mutually created plan of care within the context of assisting the person toward the higher potential of health and well-being.	Implement mutually created plan of care. Assist clients to achieve the higher potential of health and well-being.	Understanding client's present status. Understanding which interventions are appropriate and have the potential to reach higher levels of health and well-being. Understanding self as a resource to others.	Experience and competency in implementing various bio-psycho-social-spiritual interventions. Intervention skills that assist the client in achieving higher levels of health and well-being. Ability to honor and respect the client's expectations and goals.
Standard of Practice 5.5.2	*Key Concepts*	*Requisite Knowledge*	*Requisite Skills*
Holistic nurses support and promote the person's capacity for the highest level of partici-pation and problem solving in the plan of care and collaborate with other health team members when appropriate.	Support and promote client. Capacity for the highest level of participation and problem-solving. Collaboration with other health team members.	Understanding principles of how to support and promote the client's highest level of participation in care. Understanding principles of problem solving. Understanding need for collaboration with other health team members. Understanding the healing approaches of other health team members.	Ability to empower clients with knowledge and skill that promote health and well-being. Experience in facilitating client participation in care and problem solving. Ability to actively collaborate with other appropriate health care team members. Experience in resolving conflicts.

continues

Table 5–5 continued

Standard of Practice 5.5.3	*Key Concepts*	*Requisite Knowledge*	*Requisite Skills*
Holistic nurses use holistic nursing skills in implementing care including cultural competency and all ways of knowing.	Holistic nursing skills. Implementing care. Cultural competency. All ways of knowing.	Understanding bio-psycho-social-spiritual intervention strategies. Understanding principles and content involved in care that is culturally competent. Valuing right- and left-brain knowing.	Experience in implementing holistic nursing skills. Skills in implementing interventions that are consistent with the client's cultural background. Skills in implementing interventions that incorporate right- and left-brain knowing.

Standard of Practice 5.5.4	*Key Concepts*	*Requisite Knowledge*	*Requisite Skills*
Holistic nurses advocate that the person's plan, choices, and unique healing journey be honored.	Advocating for the client's plan, choices, and unique healing journey. Honoring the client's healing journey.	Understanding how to advocate for clients. Respecting and honoring the individuality and uniqueness of each client in his or her healing journey.	Ability to advocate, encourage, and uphold the client's plan, treatment choices, and individualized healing path. Skills in accepting and responding to client's expectations, choices, and goals. Ability to view health and illness as a continuum of the healing journey.

Standard of Practice 5.5.5	*Key Concepts*	*Requisite Knowledge*	*Requisite Skills*
Holistic nurses provide care that is clear about and respectful of the economic parameters of practice, balancing justice with compassion.	Care that is clear about and respects economic parameters of practice. Balancing justice with compassion.	Understanding economic constraints of client and health care agency.	Experience in implementing interventions within the context of cost and time involved.

continues

Table 5–5 continued

Standard of Practice 5.5.5	*Key Concepts*	*Requisite Knowledge*	*Requisite Skills*
		Contemplating consequences of economic restraints with need for compassionate care. Understanding the potential for abuse and conflict in care.	Skills in assessing the balance of cost versus compassion. Ability to respond to the moral and ethical challenges involved in care. Ability to recognize the economic restraints that pose threats to the client's personhood.

Nursing Activities

Within the fifth step of the holistic caring process, holistic interventions are implemented using the plan of care as the guide. Holistic nurses understand that it is the client and his or her perspective, not the nurse's, that is the focus of all caring interventions. They approach the implementation phase with a clear conviction that the client and family are active participants. Therefore, they assist in facilitating the client's highest level of participation in their care by supporting, advocating for, and honoring the client's personal goals, plan, choices, and healing journey. Holistic nurses recognize that such participation can result in client empowerment, commitment, balance, healing, and well-being.

Holistic nurses integrate human caring in all encounters with clients when implementing care. The human caring process is the "moral state in which the holistic nurse brings her or his whole self into relationship to the whole self of significant beings which reinforces the meaning and experience of oneness and unity."[5] Watson has described transpersonal human caring as the relationship between nurse and client that protects the client's vulnerability and preserves his or her humanity and dignity.[38] Caring occurs when nurses are completely receptive and respond to the needs of their clients.[39] They enter into a caring-healing relationship with an appreciation of their own wholeness and the interconnectedness they share with their clients. They support and promote the client's wholeness to facilitate harmony of body, mind, and spirit. They recognize that human beings are capable of striving toward order, self-transcendence, and transformation.[40] They honor the client's personhood and respect his or her cultural background, beliefs, and values and need for self-determination. In facilitating health and well-being, holistic nurses also appreciate that true healing is always a process of emergence into something new rather than a returning to previous states of existence.[40]

Caring interventions are not limited to curing or client recovery but rather are expanded to help clients integrate their illness experiences and transcend to new patterns of self-actualization. Although many of our clients cannot be cured of disease, they are all in need of healing. For this reason, holistic practitioners know that even during devastating crisis, illness, and death, healing can take place and growth toward wholeness can occur.[41]

Healing, however, does not follow a predictable path. The endpoint of the healing process cannot be predicted ahead of time.[40] To determine if healing has occurred, more than empirical knowing is required. Often the best method for assessing healing is the subjective knowing of both the client and the nurse. During healing encounters, there is often a sense of astonishment, reverence, and marvel. Nurses intuitively understand that something has changed, shifted, or been altered. It may be difficult or impossible to describe in words what the healing was. Both client and nurse just know that something has shifted and they trust that it is real.[40]

Holistic nurses are encouraged to refer to the interventions included in the Nursing Interventions Classification (NIC), which have been developed by a nursing team involved in the Iowa Intervention Project.[28] NIC contains an alphabetical list of over 400 interventions, each with a label, definition, detailed set of related activities that describes what it is a nurse does to implement the intervention, and list of background readings. The interventions are organized in 27 classes and 6 domains (i.e., basic physiological, complex physiological, behavioral, family, health system, safety).

It is recommended that holistic nurses use NIC, which contains all direct care interventions that nurses perform for clients including those that reflect both the independent and collaborative role of the nurse. The interventions describe treatments that nurses perform in all settings and in all specialties. The interventions focus on illness treatments, illness prevention, and health promotion. They are directed toward individuals and families, indirect care interventions (e.g., emergency cart checking), and communities (e.g., environmental management: community).

Because of its standardized language, holistic nurses use NIC to enhance the continuity of care and communication among nurses and other health care providers. It also enables them to describe their contributions to multidisciplinary health teams in achieving results.[42] Moreover, NIC has been recognized by the Joint Commission as one classification system that can be used to meet standards on uniform data.[43] The list of NANDA nursing diagnoses linked to NIC and to NOC has been developed (see NANDA Nursing Diagnosis Linked to Outcomes and Interventions, Exhibit 5–4).

Exhibit 5–4 NANDA Nursing Diagnoses Linked to Outcomes and Interventions

A. NANDA Nursing Diagnosis, Health-Seeking Behaviors

Definition

A state in which an individual in stable health is actively seeking ways to alter personal health habits and/or the environment in order to move toward a higher level of health.

Defining Characteristics

Expressed or observed desire to seek a higher level of wellness; demonstrated or observed lack of knowledge in health-promotion behaviors; stated or observed unfamiliarity with wellness community resources; expression of concern about current environmental conditions or health status; expressed or observed desire for increased control of health practice

Related Factors

To be developed

Note: Stable health states is defined as age-appropriate, illness-prevention measures achieved; client reports good or excellent health; and signs and symptoms of disease, if present, are controlled.

Source: Reprinted with permission from North American Nursing Diagnosis Association (1999). *NANDA Nursing Diagnoses: Definitions and Classification 1999–2000,* Philadelphia: NANDA.

B. Health-Seeking Behaviors Linked to Outcomes (NOC)

Definition

A state in which an individual in stable health is actively seeking ways to alter personal health habits and/or the environment in order to move toward a higher level of health.

Suggested Outcomes:

Adherence Behavior
Health Beliefs
Health Orientation
Health-Promoting Behavior
Health-Seeking Behavior

Additional Associated Outcomes:

Energy Conservation
Participation: Health Care Decisions
Psychosocial Adjustment: Life Change
Quality of Life
Risk Control
Safety Behavior: Home Physical Environment
Safety Behavior: Personal
Well-Being

Source: Reprinted with permission from M. Johnson, M. Maas, *Nursing Outcomes Classification,* p. 336, © 1977, Mosby-Year Book, Inc.

continues

Exhibit 5–4 continued

C. Health-Seeking Behaviors Linked to Interventions (NIC)

Definition

A state in which an individual in stable health is actively seeking ways to alter personal health habits and/or the environment to move toward a higher level of health.

Suggested Nursing Interventions for Problem Resolution:

Coping Enhancement
Emotional Support
Exercise Promotion
Exercise Promotion: Stretching
Family Integrity Promotion: Childbearing Family
Health Education
Health System Guidance
Immunization/Vaccination Administration
Infertility Prevention
Nutrition Management
Preconception Counseling
Self-Modification Assistance
Smoking-Cessation Assistance
Spiritual Support
Teaching: Sexuality
Weight Management

Additional Optional Interventions:

Activity Therapy
Decision-Making Support
Environmental Management: Community
Environmental Management: Worker Safety
Examination Assistance
Health Screening
Mutual Goal Setting
Reminiscence Therapy
Risk Identification
Sexual Counseling
Socialization Enhancement
Surveillance: Safety
Teaching: Individual

Source: Reprinted with permission from McCloskey and Bulechek, *Nursing Interventions Classification,* p. 636, © 1996, Mosby-Year Book, Inc.

Interventions are carried out in cooperation with other members of the health team. Holistic nurses understand the roles and healing approaches of other team members and collaborate with such members as appropriate when implementing care. Throughout this phase of the holistic caring process, nurses also are cognizant of the economic parameters imposed on the client and the health care institution and weigh the consequences of economic constraints with the need for compassionate care. In such cases, nurses must be sensitive and respond to the moral and ethical challenges involved in balancing cost versus compassion.

Holistic nurses frequently incorporate interventions that complement standard nursing care such as distraction or relaxation during painful procedures. The NIH's National Center for Complementary and Alternative Medicine has identified seven categories of therapies (Exhibit 5–5). The multitude of alternative and complementary therapies available to holistic nurses has provided additional tools to the profession. In particular, the mind/body therapies (ranging from relaxation, meditation, guided imagery, and music therapy to prayer) have become highly visible in the holistic domain primarily because such interventions provide expanded strategies that nurses can employ independently in delivering holistic, body-mind-spirit care. As a result, many of these alternative therapies increasingly are being integrated with conventional interventions as complements to caring for the client's physical illness, as well as providing clients with the understanding, meaning, and self-care strategies they need to deal with their condition to reach higher levels of health and well-being.

Exhibit 5–5 Complementary and Alternative Therapies

Classification of the National Center for Complementary and Alternative Medicine (NCCAM)

I. Alternative Systems of Medical Practice

Health care ranging from self-care according to folk principles, to care rendered in an organized health care system based on alternative traditions or practices.

Acupuncture*
Anthroposophically extended medicine
Ayurveda
Community-based health care practices
Environmental medicine
Homeopathic medicine
Latin American rural practices
Native American practices
Natural products
Naturopathic medicine
Past life therapy
Shamanism
Tibetan medicine
Traditional oriental medicine

II. Bioelectromagnetic Applications

The study of how living organisms interact with electromagnetic (EM) fields.

Blue light treatment and artificial lighting
Electroacupuncture
Electromagnetic fields
Electrostimulation and neuromagnetic stimulation devices
Magnetoresonance spectroscopy

III. Diet, Nutrition, Lifestyle Changes

The knowledge of how to prevent illness, maintain health, and reverse the effects of chronic disease through dietary or nutritional intervention.

Changes in lifestyle*
Diet†
Gerson therapy
Macrobiotics
Megavitamins
Nutritional supplements

IV. Herbal Medicine

Employing plant and plant products from folk medicine traditions for pharmacologic use.

continues

Exhibit 5–5 continued

Ginger rhizome
Echinacea (purple cornflower)
Ginkgo biloba extract
Ginseng root
Witch hazel
Wild chrysanthemum flower
Yellowdock

V. Manual Healing

Using touch and manipulation with the hands as a diagnostic and therapeutic tool.

Acupressure*
Alexander technique
Biofield therapeutics
Chiropractic medicine
Feldenkrais method
Massage therapy*
Osteopathy
Reflexology*
Rolfing®
Therapeutic touch*
Trager method
Zone therapy

VI. Mind/Body Control

Exploring the mind's capacity to affect the body, based on traditional medical systems that make use of the interconnectedness of mind and body.

Art therapy*
Biofeedback*
Counseling*,†
Dance therapy
Guided imagery*
Humor therapy
Hypnotherapy
Meditation*
Music therapy*
Prayer*
Psychotherapy
Relaxation techniques*
Support groups*
Yoga

VII. Pharmacologic and Biologic Treatments

Drugs and vaccines not yet accepted by mainstream medicine.

Antioxidizing agents
Cell treatment
Chelation therapy
Metabolic therapy
Oxidizing agents
(ozone, hydrogen peroxide)

Additional Interventions Frequently Used by Holistic Nurses†

Aromatherapy
Autogenics
Breathing exercises
Cognitive therapy
Exercise and movement
Goal setting and contracting
Healing presence
Healing touch modalities
Holistic self-assessments
Journaling
Nutrition counseling
Play therapy
Self-care interventions
Self-reflection
Smoking cessation
Weight management

Source: Compiled from B.M. Berman and D.B. Larson, Co-chairs, Editorial Review Board: *Alternative Medicine: Expanding Medical Horizons*. A Report to the National Institutes of Health on Alternative Medical Systems and Practices in the United States (Washington, DC: U.S. Government Printing Office, 1994).

*Frequently used interventions in holistic nursing practice. From B. Dossey et al., Evolving a Blueprint for Certification: Inventory of Professional Activities and Knowledge of a Holistic Nurse, *Journal of Holistic Nursing* 16, no. 1 (1998):33–56.

†Used to provide support to those experiencing situations such as addictions, death, grief, unhealthy environments, sexual abuse, and violence; to promote wellness; and to resolve relationship and lifestyle issues.

Holistic nurses understand that a primary tenet of the holistic framework centers on the concern for the wholeness and uniqueness of each individual. They understand that all interventions are holistic, not only those labeled "alternative" or "holistic," because each is capable of affecting the client's body-mind-spirit.[40] Therefore, any caring intervention that produces a physiologic change causes a corresponding psycho-social-spiritual change. Likewise, any intervention that produces a psychologic change causes a corresponding bio-social-spiritual alteration.

As a result, interventions aimed at the body (such as administering medications), the mind (such as implementing relaxation techniques), or the spirit (such as prayer), are all inherently holistic and capable of producing bio-psycho-social-spiritual outcomes.[2,40] Moreover, with clear, focused intention, the therapeutic use of self during client-nurse encounters creates change in both the client and the nurse. Adding new interventions such as alternative and complementary therapies into one's practice, however, does not make one a holistic nurse. It is the way in which the nurse incorporates the principles of holism and the process of caring that defines a holistic nurse.

All interventions that are implemented are evaluated and documented in the client's record to determine whether desired client outcomes have been achieved and to communicate the client's progress to other team members.

CASE STUDIES

1 Nurse Theresa was working with Mr. P. to prepare him for his upcoming cardiac catheterization. She reinforced the information discussed already by the cardiologist and taught the patient about the sights, sounds, smells, and physical sensations he would experience during the procedure. During the conversation, Mr. P. admitted to Theresa that he was scared to death about the cardiac catheterization. He asked if anything could be done to deal with his fear.

Theresa intently listened to the patient and his stated needs. She told him that she had encountered other patients who had felt the same way and had worked with them to develop some skills, such as relaxation and imagery, that they had successfully used to cope with their stress. She asked if he would be interested in participating in a few sessions. He said he was very interested and wanted to start immediately.

Theresa then asked Mr. P. to tell her about the most perfect, magical place that made him feel relaxed and peaceful. He described an isolated beach in Hawaii. He told her how the ocean and waves had always been a comfort to him throughout his life. Theresa related that this magical place would be perfect for his relaxation and imagery session.

Before starting the session, Theresa explained that first she would guide Mr. P. in deep breathing and relaxation and then she would weave in the information about his special beach. She explained that because it is impossible to experience fear and relaxation at the same time, he could use these skills to achieve a more relaxed state during his procedure.

Theresa guided the patient with diaphragmatic breathing and a head-to-toe relaxation script (Exhibit 5–6). She included positive imagery and role rehearsal by having him imagine what it would be like to be transported to the cardiac catheterization laboratory, what the room would look, feel, and smell like when he arrived, and what would happen as he was being prepared for the procedure. She suggested that once he was settled on the catheterization table, he would go to his special beach in Hawaii. She included images about the warmth of the sun, feel of the sand, sounds and sight of each wave coming closer to shore, the dancing of the water as it crashed into the beach, and the sight of the birds and clouds overhead. She then encouraged him to bring the beach into full, clear awareness, focusing on every detail that he could imagine—the colors, sights, feel, smells, sounds, emotions, surrounding environment, how each wave was changing, and what he might be doing.

Exhibit 5–6 General Head-to-Toe Relaxation Script

Introduction

Discuss the concept of relaxation with the patient. If the patient agrees to participate, proceed with the following:

1. Ask the patient to urinate, if necessary.
2. Dim the lights
3. Close the drapes
4. Ask the patient to remove eyeglasses or contact lenses.
5. Ask the patient to lie in a supine or semi-Fowler's position. It is sometimes helpful to place a small pillow under the knees to relieve lower back strain.

Give the patient the following instructions:

1. The purpose of the session is:
   - To relax in a wakeful state
   - To have a quiet, relaxing experience
2. First, I will guide you in a few breathing exercises to relax.
3. Then I will guide you in a head-to-toe relaxation session.
4. Then you will continue to relax for 20 minutes.
5. Now close your eyes (if you wish).
6. Find a comfortable position:
   - Hands at side of chest or on body—whatever is most comfortable
   - Legs uncrossed
7. At any time you may change positions, scratch, or swallow.
8. There may be noises around, but these will not be important if you concentrate on my voice.
9. Now think of relaxation:
   - Relax the body.
   - Relax the mind.
   - Allow yourself to let go of tension.

continues

Exhibit 5–6 continued

- Allow relaxation to happen.
- Do not strain for it, force it, or resist it.

10. I am going to guide you in relaxing.
11. To begin relaxing, take in three long, deep breaths. Breathe gently with your abdomen. This is the kind of relaxed breathing we do every night as we fall asleep. As you breathe in, let your stomach blow up like a balloon. As you exhale, let your stomach gently fall back to your spine.
12. Feel the relaxation coming over your body.
13. As you begin to relax, focus your attention on the top of your head. Let the muscles go; relax them and feel the relaxation moving in.
14. Let the relaxation flow to your forehead, temples, eyebrows, eyelids, and eyes—let go of the muscles; feel the relaxation and warmth.
15. Let the relaxation flow to your cheeks, lips, chin, and jaw:
    - Let your jaw drop down a little.
    - Let your lips part a little.
    - Let your tongue relax; just let it puddle in your mouth.
16. Relax these muscles; your whole face feels heavy, warm, and relaxed.
17. Let the relaxation flow down your throat, neck, shoulders, upper arms, elbows, lower arms, fingers, and fingertips:
    - Let these muscles hang heavy, loose, limp, and relaxed.
    - Notice how heavy and warm both arms feel; these are signs of relaxation. You might even experience a slight tingling, which is also a sign of relaxation.
18. Focus your attention on your back, spine, waist, and buttocks:
    - Smooth out these muscles, and let go of any tension.
    - Feel the relaxation and heaviness and warmth. Allow yourself to feel the bed supporting you—just let go.
19. Let the relaxation flow around to the side of your chest, abdomen, and waist; relax the muscles, and feel the relaxation, warmth, and heaviness.
20. Concentrate on your thighs, knees, calves, ankles, feet, and toes; feel how heavy your legs are, how comfortably heavy, warm, and relaxed.
21. Feel the relaxation from the top of your head to your toes:
    - Be relaxed, peacefully calm.
    - Be very quiet, silent, and relaxed.
22. Feel this relaxation flowing through your body. If there are any places in your body that are still tense, move them a little bit, and relax them.
23. Now, as you continue to relax, select a word such as the word "one" or "relax." With each exhale say the word "one" silently to yourself. Focus all of your attention on your breathing and on the word "one."
24. If a distracting thought occurs, acknowledge the passing thought. Let it go and return your concentration on your breathing and the word "one."
25. Continue this exercise for the next 20 minutes and allow the experience to relax you even more than you already are now.
26. I will be leaving the room now and will quietly come back in 20 minutes.

continues

Exhibit 5–6 continued

27. At that time, I will guide you in counting back from 5 to 1. You will come back into the room easily and quietly. You will feel very relaxed, calm, and peaceful.
28. Now continue to relax your body and your mind.

Source: Reprinted with permission from M.A. Chulay, et al., AACN *Handbook of Critical Care Nursing*, pp. 551–552, © 1997, the McGraw-Hill Companies.

Following this session, Theresa slowly guided the patient back into the room. They discussed how Mr. P. might use these techniques during his cardiac catheterization. Theresa promised to guide him in one more relaxation session before she left for the day and call the cardiac catheterization team to inform them that he would be participating in a relaxation session tomorrow. Mr. P. said he was excited about his new learned skills and believed they would be helpful to him during the procedure.

The next day following Mr. P.'s procedure, Theresa was again caring for Mr. P. He reported to her that his relaxation and imagery helped him tremendously. He commented that he saw some of the biggest waves during his catheterization that he had ever seen in his life. He stated that although some parts of the procedure were scary, he was amazed at how calm he was and how he felt he had some control over his responses to this experience.

Theresa is practicing the Standards that support implementing interventions that assist the client in achieving a higher level of health and well-being. She is receptive and responds to Mr. P.'s needs. While in a relaxed state, Theresa weaves in role rehearsal to prepare Mr. P. for the sights, sounds, and smells he will encounter. By guiding him in relaxation and imagery, she provides Mr. P. with a powerful self-care intervention that allows him to cope with his fear and fully participate in reframing his emotional responses.

2 Nurse Laetitia met two-year-old Alex and his mother, Mrs. H., when they first arrived in the day surgery preoperative holding unit. Alex was scheduled for a repeat bronchoscopy to reduce the hemangioma of his airway using laser therapy. Alex, clearly fearful, clung to his mother's skirt. Laetitia introduced herself, explained to Alex that she was his nurse and would help him get ready for his operation, and encouraged Mrs. H. to assist Alex in putting on his surgical gown and preparing him for surgery.

Mrs. H. told Laetitia that they had just moved to the area. She explained that during Alex's last bronchoscopy at an out-of-state hospital, she was given permission to gown and accompany Alex to the operating room (OR) where she was able to hold him during his anesthetic induction. She told Laetitia that because her presence had been highly successful in calming Alex and achieving a smooth anesthetic induction, she had requested permission from her new pediatric surgeon to be present again during this anesthetic induction. Mrs. H. stated that the surgeon had agreed to this plan, and she asked Laetitia about the details necessary to make it happen.

Laetitia called the OR nurse supervisor to clear the plan and was informed that family presence during anesthetic induction was against hospital policy.

The supervisor asked to talk to the patient's mother and explained that the OR rules dictated that families were not permitted in the OR. She apologized for not being able to accommodate her request but assured Mrs. H. that the preoperative medication ordered would be effective in sedating and calming Alex prior to his transport to the OR.

Within three minutes after Alex was given his preoperative oral Versed, the OR called to say they were ready. Alex disappeared behind the swinging doors kicking and screaming while his mother, now in tears, was escorted to the family waiting room.

Laetitia's care does not comply with the holistic Standards of implementing interventions because she does not recognize the significance of the mother and child's needs, nor does she value the importance to the mother of the smooth anesthetic induction for Alex that could be achieved by her presence. Perhaps because children often are transported to the OR in such fearful states or because of the standing OR rules, Laetitia does not question whether something better could be done. She does not advocate for the patient and mother's plan, choices, and unique healing journey in her discussion with the OR supervisor, nor does she question the decision when the request is denied. Her passive actions do not support a Standard of Practice that embodies holistic, family-centered care.

5.6 Evaluation

■■ Each person's responses to holistic care are regularly and systematically evaluated and the continuing holistic nature of the healing process is recognized and honored. ■■

The goal of evaluation is to determine whether the identified client outcomes have been achieved and to what extent. Three Standards of Practice demonstrate the Core Value related to evaluation of the person's responses, as described and illustrated below.

Standard of Practice 5.6.1

Holistic nurses collaborate with the person and with other health care team members when appropriate in evaluating holistic outcomes.

Standard of Practice 5.6.2

Holistic nurses explore with the person her/his understanding of the cause of any significant deviation between the responses and the expected outcomes.

Standard of Practice 5.6.3

Holistic nurses mutually create with the person and other team members a revised plan if needed.

These Standards emphasize the Core Value that holistic nurses place on partnering with the client as well as with members of the health care team in evaluating the holistic client outcomes. During this phase of the holistic caring process, the nurse and the client also collaborate in examining the possible causes or explanations for why desired outcomes were not successfully achieved. Moreover, the Standards assert that any revision of the care plan be mutually discussed and planned with the client.

Table 5–6 illustrates the nursing knowledge and skills required for a nurse to meet Standards 5.6.1, 5.6.2, and 5.6.3.

Table 5–6 Nursing Knowledge and Skills during Evaluation

Standard of Practice 5.6.1	*Key Concepts*	*Requisite Knowledge*	*Requisite Skills*
Holistic nurses collaborate with the person and with other health care team members when appropriate in evaluating holistic outcomes.	Collaborate with client. Collaborate with other members of health care team. Evaluate holistic outcomes.	Knowledge of how to evaluate outcome indicators. Knowledge of how to track the trajectory of outcome indicators. Knowledge of how to obtain quantitative and qualitative data for outcome evaluation.	Ability to compare client's current status to proposed desired outcomes to determine if end results have been achieved. Skills in collaborating with client and health team members to determine if outcomes have been achieved. Skills in using quantitative and qualitative measurement tools to evaluate outcome indicators. Skills in documenting the effectiveness of interventions on outcomes.

continues

Table 5–6 continued

Standard of Practice 5.6.2	*Key Concepts*	*Requisite Knowledge*	*Requisite Skills*
Holistic nurses explore with the person her/his understanding of the cause of any significant deviation between the responses and the expected outcomes.	Explore client's understanding of cause for deviations in expected outcomes. Deviation between actual response and expected desired outcome.	Knowledge of client's current status. Knowledge of successful outcome indicators that demonstrate desired outcomes. Ability to recognize significant deviations from desired outcome states. Valuing client's perceptions for causes of deviations from desired responses.	Proficiency in tracking trajectory of client's present state over time. Experience in evaluating gaps between present state responses and desired outcomes. Assessment and therapeutic communications skills to explore with client their understanding of significant deviations between actual responses and expected client outcomes.

Standard of Practice 5.6.3	*Key Concepts*	*Requisite Knowledge*	*Requisite Skills*
Holistic nurses mutually create with the person and other team members a revised plan if needed.	Mutually create revised care plan with client. Mutually create revised care plan with health team members.	Understanding of how to enhance health and well-being by reframing the plan of care when deviations from desired outcomes occur. Knowledge of problem-solving methods.	Expertise in bridging gaps between present state responses and desired outcomes. Ability to determine with client what actions and decisions need to be made to bridge the gap between present status and desired outcomes.

Nursing Activities

Data about the client's bio-psycho-social-spiritual responses are continuously collected and recorded throughout the holistic caring process. The information is related to the client's patterns/problems/needs, the outcome criteria, and the results of the nursing intervention. The goal of evaluation is to determine if successful client outcomes have been achieved and to what extent.

When evaluating outcomes, the nurse partners with the client to determine whether the end results have been successfully achieved. In addition, the family and other members of the health team are involved in the evaluation process. Data are gathered to evaluate the outcome indicators using quantitative and qualitative methods. For example, measurement scales from NOC are used to document the effectiveness of the specific nursing interventions in facilitating desired results. Together, the nurse, client, family, and health team members synthesize the evaluation data to determine whether successful repatterning behaviors toward wellness have occurred.[2]

During the evaluation process, clients often attain a higher level of awareness regarding previous lifestyle patterns, insight into the interconnections of all dimensions of their life, and wisdom about the benefits of repatterning behaviors. For example, case study #1 in Standard 5.2 demonstrates the insight Mrs. G. gained about the direct impact that her family, occupational, and financial stressors had on her current illness state.

Ongoing evaluation of client outcomes is necessary because of the dynamic nature of human beings and the frequent changes that occur during illness and health. Outcomes may be effectively achieved or new client outcomes may need to be developed and the plan of care revised. Factors facilitating effective outcomes or barriers preventing solutions to problems must be evaluated. Because holistic nurses highly value the client's perceptions, they recognize that clients often have insight and an intuitive understanding of what is promoting or preventing the attainment of desired end results. Thus, throughout the holistic caring process, the nurse continues to listen to the client's story and the meaning that their current situation holds for them, realizing that stories and meanings change over time.

When significant deviations from expected results occur, the nurse explores with the client the reasons or causes for such deviations, including the client's current level of motivation and commitment to move toward healing endpoints. If necessary, together the nurse and client revise the plan of care to determine which outcomes are not reasonably attainable based on the client's current perceptions and condition, are no longer consistent with the client's needs, are no longer relevant, and/or are in need of modification. This information is used to make clinical decisions about what actions need to be taken to bridge the gap between the client's present status and the desired healing state.[15]

Holistic nurses also recognize that some outcomes may not be accessible to quantitative evaluation and objective measurement. Nurses value the subjective knowing of clients in evaluating their healing journey and the success of reaching end results. They understand the significance of the clients' inner healer when patients describe that something has been shifted, altered, or changed.

The results of the outcome evaluation are documented in the client's record and any deviations from desired endpoints are noted, together with any revision in the plan of care. Such documentation is used for the purposes of communication and collaboration with the health care team as well as for research to investigate the effectiveness of specific nursing interventions on client outcomes.[44] As health care moves to outcome-based evaluations, nurses increasingly will be challenged to demonstrate the effectiveness of their interventions in achieving desired, positive, client outcomes.

CASE STUDIES

1 Nurse Renee first met Mr. B. when he was admitted to the coronary care unit (CCU) with the presumptive diagnosis of acute myocardial infarction. Prior to admission, Mr. B. had experienced severe substernal chest pain that radiated to the left shoulder, arm, and hand and was associated with nausea, vomiting, and shortness of breath. As the chief of military police at a local military base, Mr. B. stated that he worked 10 to 12 hours every day and was a hard-driving individual. He had been in excellent health before this episode and denied any previous hospitalization.

Following admission to the CCU, Mr. B. had no current chest pain and his vital signs and cardiac rhythm were stable. However, Renee assessed that the patient was highly anxious, with clenched fists and jaw, obvious muscle tension, startle reactions to minor noise, and flight of ideas with constant talking.

Renee shared these assessment findings with Mr. B. and explored whether he might be interested in participating in a relaxation and music exercise that would help him cope better with his stay in the CCU and his illness. Renee explained that the end results of relaxation and music therapy are to reduce stress and induce relaxation by a psychophysiologic quieting of body-mind-spirit. Mr. B. agreed that he was really "nervous" and was willing to try.

After providing a music history, the patient selected a soothing classical music tape from the CCU's audiocassette library. He was supplied with a tape recorder and comfortable headsets. The music was checked for the appropriate volume and turned off and the headset was placed beside the patient's pillow. A small finger thermistor was taped to the patient's left index finger and his apical heart rate and peripheral temperature were recorded. Renee guided Mr. B. with a head-to-toe relaxation script and continued with a script suggesting that Mr. B. merge his body-mind-spirit with the music. The headsets were then placed on the patient and he continued the relaxation exercise while listening to music for 20 minutes.

Following the first session, Mr. B. said that he was sure he was not doing it "right" and that he did not wish to try it again. Renee reassured Mr. B. that there was no "right" way to relax and that everyone experiences relaxation a little differently. She added that relaxation is a skill to be learned, like riding a bike, and that the more people practice the technique, the better and richer is their response. Renee encouraged the patient to continue to practice the technique a few more times before drawing any conclusions regarding its effectiveness. The patient agreed. In evaluating Mr. B.'s response to the relaxation and music, Renee observed that there had been no change in his finger temperature or heart rate following this first session.

Mr. B. was noticeably quiet following the second relaxation-music session. When Renee inquired how he perceived the session, Mr. B. said that it went OK. Again there were minimal changes in Mr. B.'s pre-post finger temperature and heart rate. Following Mr. B.'s third session, however, Renee noted an eight-degree increase in finger temperature and a 10 beat/minute decline in heart rate from pre-session readings. The patient had a small grin on his face and stated, "I can't believe what just happened to me. This stuff really works. I felt really relaxed. You know, I have a tough job. I work 10 hours a day. For me, relaxing means having a beer after work or going on a vacation one week a year. I have been walking around for 62 years with a stiff neck and I never knew it. No one ever told me how to really relax. After this [session], I know now that, when I thought I was relaxing, I really wasn't. I have never felt like this in 62 years."[45]

Renee shared with Mr. B. the increase in the peripheral temperature and decrease in heart rate that had occurred following this third session. She explained to Mr. B. that his perceived feelings and physiologic changes were all indicative of relaxation. She also explained that if Mr. B. was able to find this path that led to such psychophysiologic changes, he would be able to find it again in future sessions. She encouraged the patient to continue his sessions twice daily to assist him in coping with his hospitalization and facilitating his bio-psycho-social-spiritual recovery.

Renee made a recording of the relaxation scripts and gave it to the patient before he was transferred to the telemetry unit. Mr. B. stated that he planned to continue his music therapy sessions during the remainder of his hospitalization and after his return home. He was given catalogues on relaxing music tapes and informed that additional tapes could be purchased from the hospital's gift shop.

Renee is practicing the Standards that support evaluation of client outcomes. She understands that relaxation is an acquired skill and the effectiveness of such therapy is usually a function of practice. Thus, she was not initially concerned when Mr. B.'s first two sessions produced no measurable psychophysiologic changes. Moreover, Renee listened to the patient's story and reframed Mr. B.'s perception of doubt by explaining that the more relaxation skills are practiced, the better patients become in changing their psychophysiology. As Renee evaluated and tracked the trajectory of Mr. B's outcomes over several sessions using easily accessible CCU monitoring devices, it was clear that during the third session something changed both qualitatively and quantitatively. Mr. B. recognized that he had experienced a major shift. Renee validated this shift by sharing the changes that had occurred in the peripheral temperature and heart rate. Renee went on to frame the significance of the experience for the patient by explaining that such a shift often signifies a healing moment that can have a powerful impact on one's future perceptions, reactions, and recovery.

Renee framed the experience to empower the patient. She explained that no nurse can teach the things that Mr. B. experienced during his third session. She explained that the changes that occurred happened because of Mr. B.'s motivation, involvement, and skill—not because Renee was present. Renee understands that when patients find the path to relaxation, they are ready to continue the technique alone. Thus, supplying the patient with the relaxation tape prior to his transfer was appropriate for Mr. B.'s level of experience. Moreover, providing the patient with the opportunity to participate in the relaxation sessions assisted Mr. B. to access his inner wisdom and enhance his movement toward self-healing and health.

2 Critical Care Nurse Jill had just come on duty and was assigned to care for 12-year-old Sara, who underwent a median sternotomy for removal of a large benign mediastinal tumor two days previously. Jill introduced herself to Sara and observed that she was grimacing and breathing rapidly. When Jill asked whether Sara was having pain, Sara nodded. Jill told Sara that it was time for her pain medication, quickly returned with the methadone, and administered it to the patient.

Thirty minutes later, Jill observed that Sara was sitting in bed playing with her Gameboy. She documented in the patient's medical record that the methadone had been effective in relieving Sara's pain, as evidenced by the child's behavior.

Jill's astute observations of Sara's behavior immediately alerted her to assess Sara's level of pain. Having determined that Sara was in pain, she immediately responded to the patient's needs. Jill's actions, however, do not support the holistic Standards in evaluating patient outcomes. Pain is defined as what the patient says it is. Jill did not use a valid and reliable quantitative tool such as the FACES pain scale (i.e., on a scale of 0 to 10 with 0 indicating no pain and 10 being the worst pain one could have) to determine Sara's initial level of pain. Had she done so, she would have discovered that Sara rated her current pain as a 6. She did not collaborate with the patient to determine whether Sara wanted pain medication but rather made the clinical decision based on her assessment of behavior and respiratory rate that the patient was in need of pain relief. As a result, Sara was not included as a partner in the decision-making process.

Jill also did not collaborate with the patient to determine Sara's goals for pain management (e.g., "Sara, on a scale of 0 to 10, what do you want to say when I ask you how much you are hurting?"). Had Jill done so, she would have found out that Sara's goal for pain management was a 0 or 1 on the pain scale.

Moreover, Jill did not collaborate with the patient in evaluating the effectiveness of the pain medication following the administration of the analgesic. She assumed that Sara's behavioral manifestations (playing with her Gameboy) were a valid reflection of Sara's current level of pain, that her pain had been relieved, the intervention was effective, and the outcomes of pain management had been achieved. Had Jill used the FACES tool again to evaluate Sara's pain after the pain medication had been given, she would have learned that Sara's level of pain was still at a 4. Knowing the patient's goal for pain management (a 0 or 1) and comparing it to the patient's current level of pain (a 4) would have reframed Jill's clinical decision about pain relief, indicating that more pain medication was actually necessary to bridge the gap between the patient's present status and the desired outcome for pain control. Thus, because the outcomes for pain control were not collaborated with the patient, the nurse and patient do not have a shared outcome for their work together. Moreover, it might have been possible for Jill to introduce the patient to nonpharmacologic interventions such as deep breathing, imagery, suggestion, relaxation, or distraction as a complement to the pain management strategy.

CONCLUSION

Core Value 5, holistic caring process, is based on the universal language of the nursing process. This chapter describes what it is that holistic nurses do differently from others to transform the nursing process into the holistic caring process. These differences (in assessment, problem identification, specifying outcomes, planning and implementing care, and evaluating outcome achievement) not only reveal the application of holism to practice but also provide the criteria by which to differentiate the "good nurse" from the holistic nurse. The ability to demonstrate the congruence of these theoretical and philosophical concepts with concrete applications to each step of the holistic caring process validates the underlying assumptions of the holistic paradigm.

NOTES

1. N.C. Frisch and L.E. Frisch, *Psychiatric Mental Health Nursing: Understanding the Client as Well as the Condition* (Albany, NY: Delmar Publishers, 1998).
2. P.J. Potter and C.E. Guzzetta, "The Holistic Caring Process," in *Holistic Nursing: A Handbook for Practice*, 3d ed., eds. B.M. Dossey et al. (Gaithersburg, MD: Aspen Publishers, 2000), 315–343.
3. H.C. Erickson et al., *Modeling and Role-Modeling* (Columbia, SC: R.L. Bryan Co., 1983).
4. American Holistic Nurses' Association, *American Holistic Nurses' Association Standards of Holistic Nursing Practice* (Flagstaff, AZ: AHNA, 1998).
5. J.G. Patterson and L.T. Zderad, *Humanistic Nursing* (New York: John Wiley & Sons, 1976).
6. M.E. Doona et al., "Nursing Presence: As Real as a Milky Way Bar," *Journal of Holistic Nursing* 17, no. 1 (1999): 54–70.
7. M. McKivergin, "The Nurse as an Instrument of Healing," in *Holistic Nursing: A Handbook for Practice*, 3d ed., eds. B. Dossey et al. (Gaithersburg, MD: Aspen Publishers, 2000), 207–227.
8. C.E. Guzzetta et al., *Clinical Assessment Tools for Use with Nursing Diagnoses* (St. Louis: Mosby-Year Book, 1989), 1–40.
9. North American Nursing Diagnosis Association, Nursing Diagnoses: Definitions & Classification 1999–2000 (Philadelphia: NANDA, 1999).
10. M. Gordon, *Manual of Nursing Diagnosis* 1997–1998 (St. Louis: Mosby, 1997).
11. B.D. Schraeder and D.K. Fisher, "Using Intuitive Knowledge in the Neonatal Intensive Care Nursery," *Holistic Nursing Practice* 1, no. 3 (1987): 45–51.
12. C.E. Young, "Intuition and the Nursing Process," *Holistic Nursing Practice* 1, no. 3 (1987): 52–62.
13. L. King and J.V. Appleton, "Intuition: A Critical Review of the Research and Rhetoric," *Journal of Advanced Nursing* 26 (1997): 194–202.

14. J. Kelley, N. Frisch, and K. Avant, "A Trifocal Model of Nursing Diagnosis: Wellness Revisited," *Nursing Diagnosis* 6 (1995): 123–128.
15. D.J. Pesut and J. Herman, *Clinical Reasoning: The Art & Science of Critical and Creative Thinking* (Albany, NY: Delmar Publishers, 1999).
16. C.E. Guzzetta et al., *Clinical Assessment Tools for Use with Nursing Diagnoses* (St. Louis: Mosby-Year Book, 1989).
17. NIH Consensus Development Panel on Acupuncture, *Journal of the American Medical Association* 280, no. 17 (1998): 1518–1524.
18. B.B. Granger and M. Chulay, *Research Strategies for Clinicians* (Stamford, CT: Appleton & Lange, 1999).
19. M.A.Q. Curley, "Patient-Nurse Synergy: Optimizing Patients' Outcomes," *American Journal of Critical Care* 7, no. 1 (1998): 64–72.
20. J.C. McCloskey and G.M. Bulechek, "Classification of Nursing Intervention: Implications for Nursing Diagnoses," in *Classification of Nursing Diagnoses: Proceedings of the Tenth Conference*, eds. R.R. Carroll-Johnson and M. Paquette (Philadelphia: J.B. Lippincott Co., 1994), 116.
21. M.M. Lang and K.D. Marek, "Outcomes That Reflect Clinical Practice," in *Patient Outcomes Research: Examining the Effectiveness of Nursing Practice*, NIH Publication 93–3411 (Washington, DC: Department of Health and Human Services, 1992), 27–38.
22. American Nurses Association, Lewin-VHI, Inc., *Nursing Care Report Card for Acute Care Settings* (Washington, DC: American Nurses Publishing, 1995).
23. B.M. Jennings and N. Staggers, "The Language of Outcomes," *Advances in Nursing Science* 20, no. 4 (1998): 72–80.
24. M. Johnson and M. Maas, "The *Nursing Outcomes Classification*," *Journal of Nursing Care Quarterly* 12, no. 6 (1998): 9–20.
25. M. Johnson and M. Maas, *Nursing Outcomes Classification* (St. Louis: Mosby, 1997).
26. M. McKivergin, "The Nurse as an Instrument of Healing," in *Holistic Nursing: A Handbook for Practice*, 3d ed., eds. B. Dossey et al. (Gaithersburg, MD: Aspen Publishers, 2000), 207–212.
27. J.C. McCloskey and G.M. Bulechek, "Classification of Nursing Intervention: Implications for Nursing Diagnoses," in *Classification of Nursing Diagnoses: Proceedings of the Tenth Conference*, eds. R.R. Carroll-Johnson and M. Paquette (Philadelphia: J.B. Lippincott Co., 1994).
28. J.C. McCloskey and G.M. Bulechek, *Nursing Interventions Classification* (NIC), 2d ed. (St. Louis: Mosby, 1996).
29. B.M. Dossey and L. Keegan, "Self-Assessments: Facilitating Healing in Self and Others," in *Holistic Nursing: A Handbook for Practice*, 3d ed., eds. B.M. Dossey et al. (Gaithersburg, MD: Aspen Publishers, 2000), 361–374.
30. J.E. Engebretson and J. Headley, "Cultural Diversity and Care," in *Holistic Nursing: A Handbook for Practice*, 3d ed., eds. B.M. Dossey et al. (Gaithersburg, MD: Aspen Publishers, 2000), 283–310.
31. L. Radwin, "Conceptualizations of Decision Making in Nursing: Analytic Models and 'Knowing the Patient'," *Nursing Diagnosis* 6, no. 1 (1995): 16–22.
32. L. Radwin, "Knowing the Patient: An Empirically Generated Process Model for Individualized Interventions," *Dissertation Abstracts International* B55/01, 79 (University Microfilms, No. DA 9414164), 1994.
33. C. Tanner et al., "The Phenomenology of Knowing the Patient," *Image* 25 (1993): 273–280.

34. E. Coker, "Does Your Care Plan Tell My Story? Documenting Aspects of Personhood in Long-Term Care," *Journal of Holistic Nursing* 16, no. 4 (1998): 435–452.
35. M. McKivergin, "The Nurse as an Instrument of Healing," in *Holistic Nursing: A Handbook for Practice*, 3d ed., eds. B. Dossey et al. (Gaithersburg, MD: Aspen Publishers, 2000), 207–227.
36. S. Popkess-Vawter, "Weight Management Counseling," in *Holistic Nursing: A Handbook for Practice*, 3d ed., eds. B.M. Dossey et al. (Gaithersburg, MD: Aspen Publishers, 2000), 689–721.
37. S. Popkess-Vawter, "Weight Management Counseling," in *Holistic Nursing: A Handbook for Practice*, 3d ed., eds. B.M. Dossey et al. (Gaithersburg, MD: Aspen Publishers, 2000).
38. J. Watson, *Nursing: Human Science and Human Care* (New York: National League for Nursing Press, 1988).
39. R.C. Locsin, "Technologic Competence as Caring in Critical Care Nursing," *Holistic Nursing Practice* 12, no. 4 (1998): 50–56.
40. J.F. Quinn, "Transpersonal Human Caring and Healing," in *Holistic Nursing: A Handbook for Practice*, 3d ed., eds. B.M. Dossey et al. (Gaithersburg, MD: Aspen Publishers, 2000), 37–50.
41. M.A. Chulay, C.E. Guzzetta, and B.M. Dossey, *AACN Handbook of Critical Care Nursing* (Stamford, CT: Appleton & Lange, 1997).
42. M. Snyder et al., "Defining Nursing Interventions," *Image* 28, no. 2 (1996): 137–141.
43. http://www.nursing.uiowa.edu, Nursing Interventions Classification: Overview (1999).
44. C.E. Guzzetta, "Holistic Nursing Research," in *Holistic Nursing: A Handbook for Practice*, 3d ed., eds. B.M. Dossey et al. (Gaithersburg, MD: Aspen Publishers, 2000), 187–202.
45. C.E. Guzzetta, "Music Therapy: Hearing the Melody of the Soul," in *Holistic Nursing: A Handbook for Practice*, 3d ed., eds. B.M. Dossey et al. (Gaithersburg, MD: Aspen Publishers, 2000), 585–610.

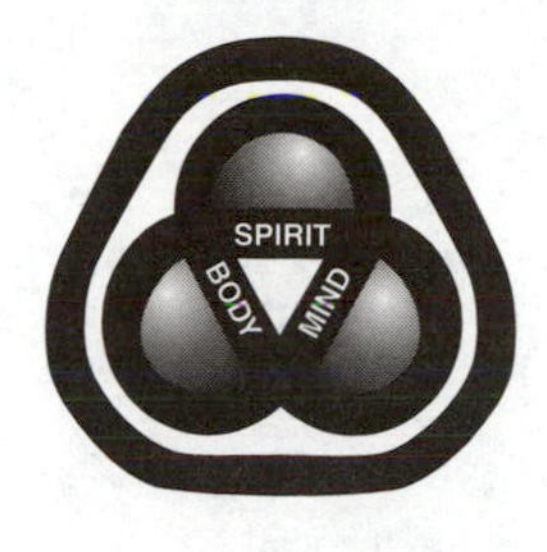

APPENDIX 5-A

HOLISTIC NURSING ASSESSMENT TOOL FOR HOSPITALIZED PATIENTS

Name: ______ Age: ______ Sex: ______
Address: ______ Telephone: ______
Significant other: ______ Telephone: ______
Date of admission: ______ Medical diagnosis: ______
Allergies: ______ Dyes: ______

	Nursing Diagnosis (Altered/High Risk for/ Potential for Enhanced)
Communicating—A pattern involving sending messages	
Read, write, understand English (circle) ______	Communication
Other language ______	Verbal
Intubated ______ Speech impaired ______	[Nonverbal]
Alternate form of communication ______	
"Valuing/Transcending"—A pattern involving spiritual growth	
Religious preference ______	[Spiritual state]
Important religious practices ______	Spiritual
Cultural orientation ______	well-being
Cultural practices ______	Spiritual distress
Meaning and purpose in life ______	Hopelessness
Inner strengths ______	Powerlessness
Interconnections (self, others, universe, higher power) ______	
Relating—A pattern involving establishing bonds	
[Alterations in role]	
Marital status ______	[Role performance]
Age and health of significant other ______	Parenting
	Sexuality patterns
Number of children ______ Ages ______	
Responsibilities in home ______	
Financial support ______	Family processes
Occupation ______	
Job satisfaction/concerns ______	
Physical/mental energy expenditures ______	
Sexual relationships (satisfactory/unsatisfactory) ______	
Physical difficulties related to sex ______	

Source: Adapted with permission from C.E. Guzzetta, S.D. Bunton, L.A. Prinkey, A.P. Sherer, and P.C. Seifert, *Clinical Assessment Tools for Use with Nursing Diagnoses,* pp. 15–22, © 1989, Mosby-Year Book, Inc.; Revised 1999.

	Nursing Diagnosis (Altered/High Risk for/ Potential for Enhanced)
[Alterations in socialization]	
Quality of relationships with others ______	
Patient's description ______	Impaired social interaction
Significant other's description ______	
Staff observations ______	
Verbalizes feelings of being alone ______	Loneliness
Attributed to ______	Social isolation
Knowing—A pattern involving the meaning associated with information	
Previous hospitalization/surgeries ______	
______	Knowledge deficit
Educational level ______	
History of the following diseases:	
Heart ______	
Lung ______	
Liver ______ Kidney ______	
Cerebrovascular ______ Rheumatic fever ______	
Thyroid ______	
Diabetes ______	
Medication ______	
Current health problems ______	
______	
Current medications ______	
______	

Risk factors	Present	Knowledge of	
1. Hypertension	______	______	
2. Hyperlipidemia	______	______	
3. Smoking	______	______	
4. Obesity	______	______	
5. Diabetes	______	______	
6. Sedentary living	______	______	
7. Stress	______	______	
8. Alcohol use	______	______	
9. Oral contraceptives	______	______	Altered family process: Alcoholism
10. Family history ______			

______	
Knowledge of planned test/surgery ______	
______	
Misconceptions ______	
Readiness to learn ______	[Learning]
Learning impeded by ______	Thought processes
Feeling—A pattern involving the subjective awareness of information	
[Alterations in comfort]	
Pain/discomfort	
Onset ______ Duration ______	
Location ______ Quality ______ Radiation ______	Pain
Associated factors ______	Chronic
Aggravating factors ______	[Acute]

	Nursing Diagnosis (Altered/High Risk for/ Potential for Enhanced)
Alleviating factors ______	[Discomfort] Chronic, Acute
[Alterations in emotional integrity]	
Recent stressful life events ______	Anxiety
Verbalizes feelings of fear or anxiety ______	Chronic sorrow
Source ______	Nausea
Physical manifestations ______	Fear
	Post-trauma response
Moving—A pattern involving activity	Rape-trauma syndrome
[Alterations in activity]	
History of physical disability ______	Impaired physical mobility
Limitations in daily activities ______	Activity intolerance
	Fatigue
Exercise habits ______	Impaired walking
[Alterations in rest]	Impaired bed mobility
Hours slept/night ______ Difficulties ______	Impaired transfer ability
Sleep aids (pillows, medications, food) ______	
[Alterations in recreation]	Sleep pattern disturbance
Leisure activities ______	
Social activities ______	Sleep deprivation
[Alterations in activities of daily living]	
Home maintenance management ______	Deficit in diversional activity
Size and arrangement of home (stairs, bathroom) ______	
Housekeeping responsibilities ______	Impaired home maintenance management
Shopping responsibilities ______	
Health maintenance	
Health insurance ______	
Regular physical checkups ______	Health maintenance
[Alterations in self-care]	Adult failure to thrive
Ability to perform ADL:	Self-care
Independent ______ Dependent ______	Feeding
Specify deficits ______	Bathing
Discharge planning needs ______	Dressing
	Toileting
Perceiving—A pattern involving the reception of information	Delayed surgical recovery
[Alterations in self-concept]	
Patient's description of himself/herself ______	
Effects of illness/surgery on self-concept ______	Body image
	Self-esteem
[Sensory/perceptual alterations]	Personal identity
Vision impaired ______ Glasses ______	
Visual examination ______	Visual
Auditory impaired ______ Hearing aid ______	
Auditory examination ______	Auditory
Kinesthetics impaired ______ Romberg ______	

Gustatory impaired ____________________

Tactile impaired ____________ Examination ____________

Olfactory impaired ____________ Examination ____________

Reflexes: Biceps R ___ L ___ Triceps R ___ L ___

Brachio-radialis R ___ L ___ Knee R ___ L ___

Ankle R ___ L ___ Plantar R ___ L ___

Choosing—A pattern involving the selection of alternatives

[Alterations in coping]

Patient's usual problem-solving methods ____________________

Family's usual problem-solving methods ____________________

Patient's method of dealing with stress ____________________

Family's method of dealing with stress ____________________

Patient's affect ____________________

Physical manifestations ____________________

[Alterations in participation]

Compliance with past/current health care regimen ____________________

Willingness to comply with future health care regimen ____________________

Exchanging—A pattern involving mutual giving and receiving

[Alterations in nutrition]

Teeth, gums, lesions ____________________

Dentures ____________________

Ideal body weight ____________________

Height ____________ Weight ____________

Eating patterns

Number of meals per day ____________________

Special diet ____________________

Where eaten ____________________

Food preferences/intolerances ____________________

Food allergies ____________________

Caffeine intake (coffee, tea, soft drinks) ____________________

Appetite changes ____________________

Presence of nausea/vomiting ____________________

Current therapy

NPO ____________ NG suction ____________

Tube feeding ____________________

TPN ____________________

Laboratory results

Na ________ K ________ Cl ________ Glucose ________

Cholesterol ________ Triglycerides ________ Fasting ________

Nursing Diagnosis
(Altered/High Risk for/
Potential for Enhanced)

Kinesthetic
Gustatory
Tactile
Olfactory
Reflexes

Ineffective individual coping
Ineffective family coping

Noncompliance
Ineffective management of therapeutic regimen
Family
Individual
Community

Altered dentition
Oral mucous membrane
Altered nutrition
More than body requirements

Less than body requirements

Nausea

[Alterations in physical regulation]

[Immune]

Lymph nodes enlarged__________ Location ____________________

WBC count ____________________ Differential ____________________

Alteration in body temperature

Temperature____________________ Route____________________

[Alterations in physical integrity]

Skin integrity __________ Rashes ____________ Lesions ____________

Petechiae________________ Surgical incision ____________________

Bruising________________ Abrasions ____________________

[Alterations in circulation]

Cerebral (circle appropriate response)

Pupils	Eye opening
L 2 3 4 5 6 mm	None (1)
R 2 3 4 5 6 mm	To pain (2)
Reaction: Brisk ________________	To speech (3)
Sluggish ____________________	Spontaneous (4)
Nonreactive ________________	

Best verbal	Best motor
Intubated (0)	Flaccid (1)
Mute (1)	Extensor response (2)
Incomprehensible sound (2)	Flexor response (3)
Inappropriate words (3)	Semipurposeful (4)
Confused conversation (4)	Localized to pain (5)
Oriented (5)	Obeys commands (6)

Glasgow coma scale total

____

Neurological changes/symptoms ____________________

[Cardiac]

Apical rate and rhythm ____________________

PMI ____________________

Heart sounds/murmurs ____________________

Dysrhythmias ____________________

Pacemaker ____________________

BP:	Sitting	Lying	Standing
	R _____ L _____	R _____ L _____	R _____ L _____

A-Line reading ____________________

Cardiac index ____________________ Cardiac output ________________

CVP ___________PAP ___________ PCWP ____________________

IV fluids ____________________

IV cardiac medications ____________________

____

Serum enzymes ____________________

Peripheral

Pulses: A = absent B = bruits D = Doppler

+ 3 = bounding + 2 = palpable + 1 = faintly palpable

Carotid	R ____ L ____	Popliteal	R ____ L ____
Brachial	R ____ L ____	Posterior tibial	R ____ L ____

Nursing Diagnosis
(Altered/High Risk for/
Potential for Enhanced)

Infection
Hypothermia
Hyperthermia
Ineffective thermoregulation
Impaired skin integrity
Impaired tissue integrity
Latex allergy response

Cerebral tissue perfusion

Fluid volume
Deficit
Excess
Imbalance

Cardiac output

Confusion
Impaired memory

Cardiopulmonary tissue perfusion

Fluid volume
Deficit
Excess

Cardiac output

Peripheral tissue perfusion
Peripheral neurovascular dysfunction

Radial R ____ L ____ Dorsalis pedis R ____ L ____
Femoral R ____ L ____
Jugular venous distention R ____ L ____
Skin temperature__________ Color______________________________
Edema __________ Capillary refill ______________________________
Clubbing _________ Claudication ______________________________
Gastrointestinal
Liver: Enlarged ____________ Ascites ______________________________
Renal
Urine output: 24 hour _______________ Average hourly ___________
BUN ______________ Creatinine ______________ Specific gravity _____
Urine studies ____
[Alterations in oxygenation]
Rate ______________ Rhythm __________ Depth __________________
Labored/unlabored (circle) Chest expansion ___________________________
Use of accessory muscles____
Orthopnea ____
Breath sounds ____
Complaints of dyspnea ________________ Precipitated by ____________
Cough: Productive/nonproductive ____________________________________
Sputum: Color ____________ Amount _____________ Consistency _______
LOC _______________ Splinting ________________________________
Arterial blood gases/O_2 sat.___________________________________
Oxygen percent and device ___________________________________
Ventilator ____
[Alterations in elimination]
Bowel
Abdominal physical examination ___________________________________
Usual bowel habits ____
Alterations from normal_______________________________________
Urinary
Bladder distention ____
Color ________________________ Catheter ________________________
Usual urinary pattern _______________________________________
Alterations from normal_______________________________________

Nursing Diagnosis
(Altered/High Risk for/ Potential for Enhanced)

Fluid volume
Deficit
Excess
Imbalance
Cardiac output

GI tissue perfusion

Renal tissue perfusion

Fluid volume
Cardiac output

Ineffective airway clearance
Ineffective breathing patterns
Ineffective gas exchange
Inability to sustain spontaneous ventilation

Dysfunctional ventilatory weaning response
Bowel patterns
Constipation
Diarrhea
Incontinence
Urinary patterns
Incontinence
Retention

ADL = activities of daily living; A-line = arterial line; BP = blood pressure; BUN = blood urea nitrogen; CVP = central venous pressure; GI = gastrointestinal; IV = intravenous; LOC = level of consciousness; NG = nasogastric; NPO = nothing by mouth; PAP = pulmonary artery pressure; PCWP = pulmonary capillary wedge pressure; PMI = point of maximal impulse; TPN = total parenteral nutrition

Energy Field Patterns

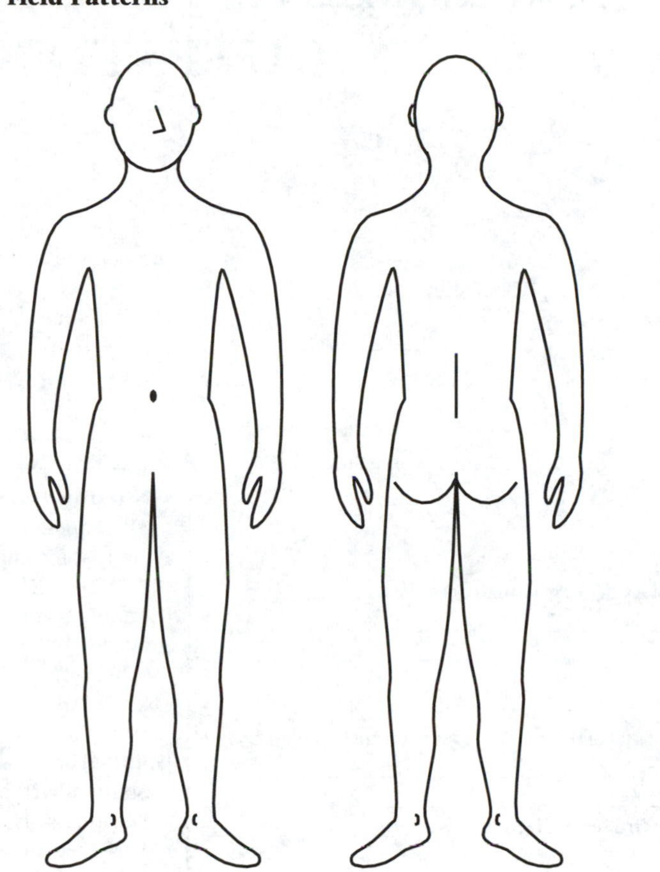

Nursing Diagnosis
(Altered/High Risk for/
Potential for Enhanced)

Energy field
disturbance

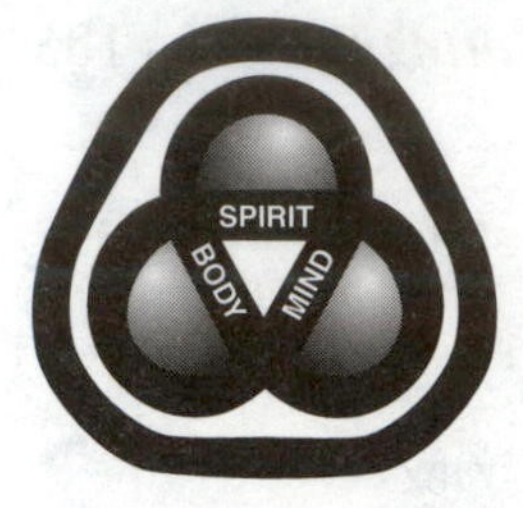

APPENDIX 5-B

HOLISTIC NURSING ASSESSMENT TOOL FOR OUTPATIENTS

Name: ______________________ Age: ________ Sex: ________
Address: ______________________ Telephone: ________
Significant other: ______________________ Telephone: ________
Date of admission: ______________________ Medical diagnosis: ________
Allergies: ______________________ Dyes: ________

	Nursing Diagnosis (Altered/High Risk for/ Potential for Enhanced)
Communicating—A pattern involving sending messages Verbal: ________ Nonverbal: ________	[Communication, altered] Verbal Nonverbal
"Valuing/Transcending"—A pattern involving spiritual growth Meaning and Purpose in Life: ________ Inner Strengths: ________ Interconnections (Self, Others, Universe, Higher Power): ________	[Spiritual State] Spiritual well-being Spiritual distress Hopelessness Powerlessness
Relating—A pattern involving establishing bonds Role (Marital Status, Children, Parents): ________ Occupation: ________ Sexual Relationships: ________ Socialization: ________	Role performance, altered Parenting, altered Parental role conflict [Work] Sexual dysfunction Family process, altered Sexuality patterns, altered [Socialization, altered] Social interaction, impaired Social isolation Loneliness

Source: Adapted with permission from C.E. Guzzetta, S.D. Bunton, L.A. Prinkey, A.P. Sherer, and P.C. Seifert, *Clinical Assessment Tools for Use with Nursing Diagnoses*, pp. 15–22, © 1989, Mosby-Year Book, Inc.; Revised 1999.

	Nursing Diagnosis (Altered/High Risk for/ Potential for Enhanced)
Knowing—A pattern involving the meaning associated with information	
Orientation: ______	Thought processes, altered
	[Orientation]
	Confusion
Memory: ______	Impaired memory
Previous Illnesses/Hospitalizations/Surgeries: ______	
Identified Health Problems (Present/History): ______	
Current Medications (Medication Allergies): ______	
Risk Factors (Smoking, Family History, etc.): ______	Altered family process
	Alcoholism
Perception/Knowledge of Health/Illness: ______	Knowledge deficit (Specify)
Expectations of Holistic Health Intervention: ______	
Readiness to Learn (Ready, Willing, Able): ______	[Learning]
Feeling—A pattern involving the subjective awareness of information	
Comfort: ______	[Comfort, altered]
	Pain, chronic
	Pain, acute
	[Discomfort, chronic]
	[Discomfort, acute]
	Nausea
Emotional Integrity States: ______	[Grieving]
	Anticipatory
	Dysfunctional
	Anxiety
	Fear
	[Anger]
	[Guilt]
	[Shame]
	[Sadness]
	Chronic sorrow
	Post-trauma response
	Rape-trauma syndrome
Moving—A pattern involving activity	
Activity (Physical Mobility Limitations): ______	[Activity, altered]
	Activity intolerance
	Impaired physical mobility

Rest: ______________________________

Recreation: ______________________________

Environmental Maintenance: ______________________________

Health Maintenance: ______________________________

Self-Care: ______________________________

Perceiving—A pattern involving the reception of information

Sensory Perception: ______________________________

Self-Concept: ______________________________

Nursing Diagnosis
(Altered/High Risk for/
Potential for Enhanced)

Impaired walking
Impaired transfer mobility
Fatigue
Sleep pattern disturbance
Sleep deprivation
[Hypersomnia]
[Insomnia]
[Nightmares]
Diversional activity deficit
Impaired home maintenance management
[Safety hazards]
Health maintenance, altered
Adult failure to thrive
Bathing/hygiene deficit
Dressing/grooming deficit
Feeding deficit
Toileting deficit
Delayed surgical recovery

[Sensory perception, altered]
Visual
Auditory
Kinesthetic
Gustatory
Tactile
Olfactory
Unilateral neglect
[Self-concept, altered]
Body image disturbance
Personal identity disturbance
Self-esteem disturbance
—Chronic low
—Situational

	Nursing Diagnosis (Altered/High Risk for/ Potential for Enhanced)
Choosing—A pattern involving the selection of alternatives	
Coping:	Individual coping, ineffective
	Adjustment: impaired
Judgment/Decisions:	Conflict: decisional
	Coping: defensive
	Denial: impaired
Participation:	Noncompliance
Family Coping:	[Family coping, ineffective]
	Compromised
	Disabled
	Ineffective management of therapeutic regimen
	Family
	Individual
	Community
Exchanging—A pattern involving mutual giving and receiving	
Nutrition:	[Nutrition, altered]
	[Nutritional deficit]
	< or > Body requirements
	Oral mucous membranes, impaired
	Altered dentition
	Nausea
Elimination:	[Bowel elimination, altered]
	Bowel incontinence
	Constipation: colonic
	Constipation: perceived
	Diarrhea
	GI tissue perfusion
Renal/Urinary:	[Urinary elimination, altered]
	Incontinence (specify)
	Retention
	[Enuresis]
	Renal tissue perfusion
Physical/Tissue Integrity:	[Tissue integrity, impaired]
	Impaired skin integrity
	Latex allergy response

	Nursing Diagnosis (Altered/High Risk for/ Potential for Enhanced)
______	[Injury: Risk]
______	Aspiration
______	Disuse syndrome
______	Poisoning
______	Suffocation
Physical Regulation: ______	Trauma
Immune: ______	[Physical regulation, altered]
______	Infection: risk
______	Altered protection
______	Thermoregulation, ineffective
______	—Hypothermia
Circulation: ______	—Hyperthermia
______	Cardiac output, decreased
______	[Tissue perfusion, altered]
______	Cardiopulmonary
______	Cerebral
______	Peripheral
______	[Fluid volume, altered]
______	Deficit
______	Deficit: risk
______	Excess
______	Imbalance
Oxygenation: ______	[Respiration, altered]
______	Airway clearance, ineffective
______	Breathing pattern, ineffective
______	Gas exchange, impaired
Hormonal/Metabolic Patterns: ______	[Menstrual patterns]
______	[Premenstrual syndrome]
______	
______	

Energy Field Patterns

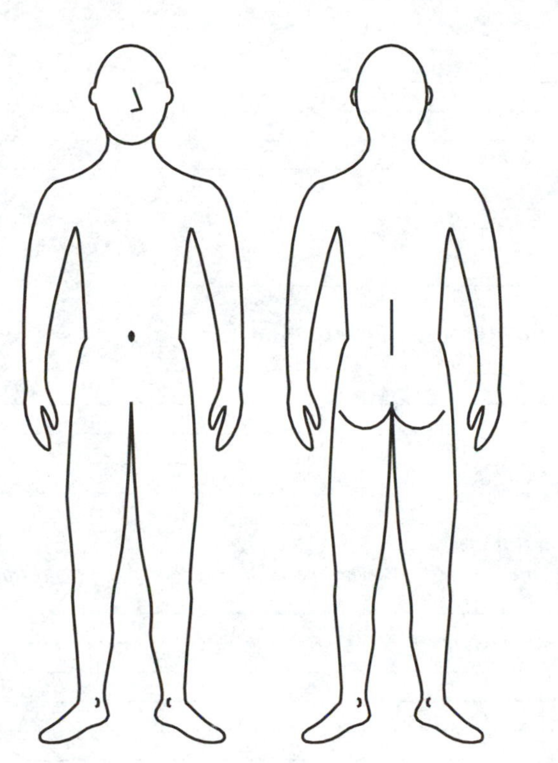

Nursing Diagnosis
(Altered/High Risk for/
Potential for Enhanced)

Energy field
disturbance

ADDITIONAL COMMENTS:

____
____
____
____
____
____
____
____

Goals

1. ____
2. ____
3. ____
4. ____
5. ____

Prioritized Nursing Diagnosis/Problem List/Theory-Based Plan of Care **Date**

1. ______________________________ ____________
2. ______________________________ ____________
3. ______________________________ ____________
4. ______________________________ ____________
5. ______________________________ ____________

Signature ______________________________ Date ____________

Holistic Nursing Care Plan

Name: ______________________________

Date: ______________________________

Client Goals:

1. ______________________________
2. ______________________________
3. ______________________________
4. ______________________________

Nursing Diagnosis and Related Factors	*Client/Patient Outcomes Outcome Criteria*	*Therapeutic Intervention*	*Evaluation*

Client Signature ______________________________

Date ______________________________

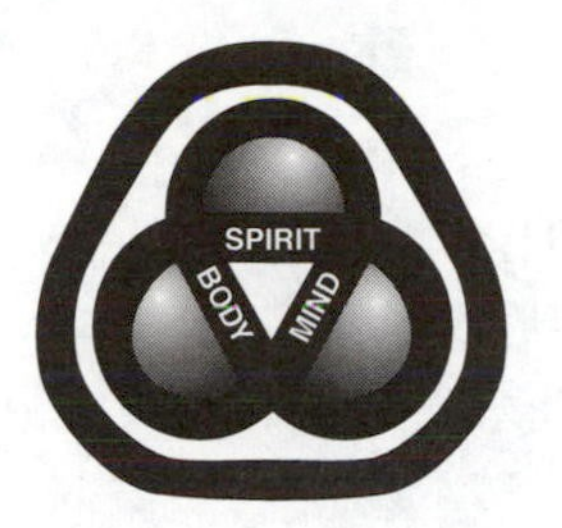

APPENDIX A

SELF-ASSESSMENT TOOL

The **AHNA Standards of Holistic Nursing Practice** can serve as a self-assessment tool to explore your knowledge base and the integration of the standards in your clinical practice, research, and personal self-care. The blueprint of this tool follows the five Core Values contained within the AHNA Standards:

Core Value 1. Holistic Philosophy and Education
Core Value 2. Holistic Ethics, Theories, and Research
Core Value 3. Holistic Nurse Self-Care
Core Value 4. Holistic Communication, Therapeutic Environment, and Cultural Diversity
Core Value 5. Holistic Caring Process

Instructions:

Take the time now to complete your self-assessment. Under each AHNA Core Value are Standards of Practice. A Standard of Practice is a group of statements describing the expected level of care by a holistic nurse. Rate these task statements for the importance of the knowledge (Column #I) and for the frequency of performance (Column #II). Use a ruler on the correct line. At 3, 6, 9, and 12 months, again repeat your self-assessment and check your increased levels of knowledge and frequency of activity.

Column #I—Knowledge: Using this scale, indicate how important each statement is to your knowledge base as a holistic nurse:

Not important: This knowledge is ***not*** required for me to practice holistic nursing.
Slightly important: This knowledge is required ***from time to time,*** but my performance could be acceptable without it.
Important: This knowledge is ***generally*** required in order for me to perform satisfactorily as a holistic nurse. Without it, my performance could be marginal.
Very important: This knowledge is ***one of the key*** requirements for my work in holistic nursing.

Place a check in the appropriate box that corresponds to your rating as to the importance of knowledge in Column #I.

Column #II—Frequency: Using the following scale, select the response that most closely matches the number of times a week you perform the activity:

Do Not Perform
Perform Less Than Once Per Week
Perform 1–5 Times Per Week
Perform 6–10 Times Per Week
Perform Greater Than 10 Times Per Week

Place a check in the appropriate box beside each activity to indicate how frequently you perform the activities each week.

Column #III—Progress Report: Check off your progress at 3 months, 6 months, 9 months, and 12 months.

	Where I Want to Be									Check off where you have improved			
	Date:												
	I Knowledge				II Frequency of Activity					III Progress Report			
	Not important	Slightly important	Important	Very important	Do not perform	Less than 1 per week	1–5 per week	6–10 per week	Greater than 10 per week	3 Months	6 Months	9 Months	12 Months
CORE VALUE 1. HOLISTIC PHILOSOPHY AND EDUCATION **1.1 Holistic Philosophy:** Holistic nurses develop and expand their conceptual framework and overall philosophy in the art and science of holistic nursing to model, practice, teach, and conduct research in the most effective manner possible.													
Standards of Practice Holistic nurses: 1.1.1 recognize the person's capacity for self-healing and the importance of supporting the natural development and unfolding of that capacity.													
1.1.2 support, share, and recognize expertise and competency in holistic nursing practice that is used in many diverse clinical and community settings.													
1.1.3 participate in person-centered care by being a partner, coach, and mentor who actively listens and supports others in reaching personal goals.													
1.1.4 focus on strategies to bring harmony, unity, and healing to the nursing profession.													
1.1.5 communicate with traditional health care practitioners about appropriate referrals to other holistic practitioners when needed.													
1.1.6 interact with professional organizations in a leadership or membership capacity at local, state, national, and international levels to further expand the knowledge and practice of holistic nursing and awareness of holistic health issues.													

	Where I Want to Be Date:									Check off where you have improved			
	I Knowledge				II Frequency of Activity					III Progress Report			
	Not important	Slightly important	Important	Very important	Do not perform	Less than 1 per week	1–5 per week	6–10 per week	Greater than 10 per week	3 Months	6 Months	9 Months	12 Months
1.2 Holistic Education: Holistic nurses acquire and maintain current knowledge and competency in holistic nursing practice.													
Standards of Practice Holistic nurses: 1.2.1 participate in activities of continuing education and related fields that have relevance to holistic nursing practice.													
1.2.2 identify areas of knowledge from nursing and various fields such as biomedicine, epidemiology, behavioral medicine, cultural and social theories.													
1.2.3 continually develop and standardize holistic nursing guidelines, protocols, and practice to promote competency in holistic nursing practice and ensure quality of care to individuals.													
1.2.4 use the results of quality care activities to initiate change in holistic nursing practice.													
1.2.5 may seek certification in holistic nursing as one means of advancing the philosophy and practice of holistic nursing.													
CORE VALUE 2. HOLISTIC ETHICS, THEORIES, AND RESEARCH **2.1 Holistic Ethics:** Holistic nurses hold to a professional ethic of caring and healing that seeks to preserve wholeness and dignity of self, students, colleagues, and the person who is receiving care in all practice settings, be it in health promotion, birthing centers, acute or chronic care facilities, end-of-life centers, or homes.													

	Where I Want to Be — Date:									Check off where you have improved			
	I Knowledge				II Frequency of Activity					III Progress Report			
	Not important	Slightly important	Important	Very important	Do not perform	Less than 1 per week	1–5 per week	6–10 per week	Greater than 10 per week	3 Months	6 Months	9 Months	12 Months
Standards of Practice Holistic nurses: 2.1.1 identify the ethics of caring and its contribution to unity of self, others, nature, and God/Life Force/Absolute/Transcendent as central to holistic nursing practice.													
2.1.2 integrate the standards of holistic nursing practice with applicable state laws and regulations governing nursing practice.													
2.1.3 engage in activities that respect, nurture, and enhance the integral relationship with the earth, and advocate for the well-being of the global community's economy, education, and social justice.													
2.1.4 advocate for the rights of patients to have educated choices into their plan of care.													
2.1.5 participate in peer evaluation to ensure knowledge and competency in holistic nursing practice.													
2.1.6 protect the personal privacy and confidentiality of individuals, especially with health care agencies and managed care organizations.													
2.2 Holistic Theories: Holistic nurses recognize that holistic nursing theories provide the framework for all aspects of holistic nursing practice and transformational leadership.													
Standards of Practice Holistic nurses: 2.2.1 strive to use nursing theories to develop holistic nursing practice and transformational leadership.													
2.2.2 interpret, use, and document information relevant to a person's care according to a theoretical framework.													

	Where I Want to Be Date:												Check off where you have improved
	I Knowledge				II Frequency of Activity					III Progress Report			
	Not important	Slightly important	Important	Very important	Do not perform	Less than 1 per week	1–5 per week	6–10 per week	Greater than 10 per week	3 Months	6 Months	9 Months	12 Months
2.3 Holistic Nursing and Related Research: Holistic nurses provide care and guidance to persons through nursing interventions and holistic therapies consistent with research findings and other sound evidence.													
Standards of Practice Holistic nurses: 2.3.1 use available research and evidence from different explanatory models to mutually create a plan of care with a person.													
2.3.2 use expert clinical judgment to select appropriate interventions.													
2.3.3 discuss holistic application to clinical situations where rigorous research has not been done.													
2.3.4 create an environment conducive to systematic inquiry into healing and health issues by engaging in research or supporting and utilizing the research of others.													
2.3.5 disseminate research findings at meetings and through publications to further develop the foundation and practice of holistic nursing.													
2.3.6 provide consultation services on holistic nursing interventions to persons and communities based on research.													
CORE VALUE 3. HOLISTIC NURSE SELF-CARE **3.1 Holistic Nurse Self-Care:** Holistic nurses engage in self-care and further develop their own personal awareness of being an instrument of healing to better serve self and others.													

	Where I Want to Be Date:									Check off where you have improved			
	I Knowledge				II Frequency of Activity					III Progress Report			
	Not important	Slightly important	Important	Very important	Do not perform	Less than 1 per week	1–5 per week	6–10 per week	Greater than 10 per week	3 Months	6 Months	9 Months	12 Months
Standards of Practice Holistic nurses: 3.1.1 recognize that a person's body-mind-spirit has healing capacities that can be enhanced and supported through self-care practices.													
3.1.2 identify and integrate self-care strategies to enhance their physical, psychological, sociological, and spiritual well-being.													
3.1.3 recognize and address at-risk health patterns and begin the process of change.													
3.1.4 consciously cultivate awareness and understanding about the deeper meaning, purpose, inner strengths, and connections with self, others, nature, and God/Life Force/Absolute/Transcendent.													
3.1.5 use clear intention to care for self and to seek a sense of balance, harmony, and joy in daily life.													
3.1.6 participate in the evolutionary holistic process with the understanding that crisis creates opportunity in any setting.													
CORE VALUE 4. HOLISTIC COMMUNICATION, THERAPEUTIC ENVIRONMENT, AND CULTURAL DIVERSITY **4.1 Holistic Communication:** Holistic nurses engage in holistic communication to ensure that each person experiences the presence of the nurse as authentic and sincere; there is an atmosphere of shared humanness that includes a sense of connectedness and attention reflecting the individual's uniqueness.													

	Where I Want to Be Date:									Check off where you have improved			
	I Knowledge				II Frequency of Activity					III Progress Report			
	Not important	Slightly important	Important	Very important	Do not perform	Less than 1 per week	1–5 per week	6–10 per week	Greater than 10 per week	3 Months	6 Months	9 Months	12 Months
Standards of Practice Holistic nurses: 4.1.1 develop an awareness of the most frequently encountered challenges to holistic communication.													
4.1.2 increase therapeutic and cultural competence skills to enhance their effectiveness through listening to themselves and others.													
4.1.3 explore with each person those strategies that can assist her/him, as desired, to understand the deeper meaning, purpose, inner strengths, and connections with self, others, nature, and God/Life Force/Absolute/Transcendent.													
4.1.4 recognize that holistic communication and awareness of individuals is a continuously evolving multi-level exchange that offers itself through dreams, images, symbols, sensations, meditations, and prayers.													
4.1.5 respect the person's health trajectory, which may be incongruent with conventional wisdom.													
4.2 Therapeutic Environment: Holistic nurses recognize that each person's environment includes everything that surrounds the individual, both the external and internal (physical, mental, emotional, and spiritual), as well as patterns not yet understood.													
Standards of Practice Holistic nurses: 4.2.1 promote environments conducive to experiencing healing, wholeness, and harmony, and care for the person in as healthy an environment as possible.													

	Where I Want to Be Date:													Check off where you have improved
	I Knowledge				II Frequency of Activity					III Progress Report				
	Not important	Slightly important	Important	Very important	Do not perform	Less than 1 per week	1–5 per week	6–10 per week	Greater than 10 per week	3 Months	6 Months	9 Months	12 Months	
4.2.2 work toward creating organizations that value sacred space and environments that enhance healing.														
4.2.3 integrate holistic principles, standards, policies, and procedures in relation to environmental safety and emergency preparedness.														
4.2.4 recognize that the well-being of the ecosystem of the planet is a prior determining condition for the well-being of the human.														
4.2.5 promote social networks and social environments where healing can take place.														
4.3 Cultural Diversity: Holistic nurses recognize each person as a whole being of body-mind-spirit and mutually create a plan of care consistent with cultural backgrounds, health beliefs, sexual orientation, values, and preferences.														
Standards of Practice Holistic nurses: 4.3.1 assess and incorporate the person's cultural practices, values, beliefs, meaning of health, illness, and risk behaviors in care and health education.														
4.3.2 use appropriate community resources and experts to extend their understanding of different cultures.														
4.3.3 assess for discriminatory practices and change as necessary.														
4.3.4 identify discriminatory health care practices as they impact the person and engage in effective nondiscriminatory practices.														

CORE VALUE 5. HOLISTIC CARING PROCESS

	Where I Want to Be Date:									Check off where you have improved			
	I Knowledge				II Frequency of Activity					III Progress Report			
	Not important	Slightly important	Important	Very important	Do not perform	Less than 1 per week	1–5 per week	6–10 per week	Greater than 10 per week	3 Months	6 Months	9 Months	12 Months
5.1 Assessment: Each person is assessed holistically using appropriate traditional and holistic methods while the uniqueness of the person is honored.													
Standards of Practice Holistic nurses: 5.1.1 use an assessment process including appropriate traditional and holistic methods to systematically gather information.													
5.1.2 value all types of knowing including intuition when gathering data from a person and validate this intuitive knowledge with the person when appropriate.													
5.2 Patterns/Problems/Needs: Each person's actual and potential patterns/problems/needs and life processes related to health, wellness, disease, or illness that may or may not facilitate well-being are identified and prioritized.													
Standards of Practice Holistic nurses: 5.2.1 assist the person to access inner wisdom that can provide opportunities to enhance and support growth, development, and movement toward health and well-being.													
5.2.2 collect data and collaborate with the person and health care team members as appropriate to identify and record a list of actual and potential patterns/problems/needs.													
5.2.3 use collected data to formulate an etiology of the person's identified actual or potential patterns/problems/needs.													
5.2.4 make referrals to other holistic practitioners or traditional therapist when appropriate.													

	Where I Want to Be — Date:									Check off where you have improved			
	I Knowledge				II Frequency of Activity					III Progress Report			
	Not important	Slightly important	Important	Very important	Do not perform	Less than 1 per week	1–5 per week	6–10 per week	Greater than 10 per week	3 Months	6 Months	9 Months	12 Months
5.3 Outcomes: Each person's actual or potential patterns/problems/needs have appropriate outcomes specified.													
Standards of Practice Holistic nurses: 5.3.1 honor the person in all phases of her/his healing process regardless of expectations or outcomes.													
5.3.2 identify and partner with the person to specify measurable outcomes and realistic goals.													
5.4 Therapeutic Care Plan: Each person engages with the holistic nurse to mutually create an appropriate plan of care that focuses on health promotion, recovery, restoration, or peaceful dying so that the person is as independent as possible.													
Standards of Practice Holistic nurses: 5.4.1 partner with the person in a mutual decision process to create a health care plan for each pattern/problem/need or opportunity to enhance health and well-being.													
5.4.2 help a person identify areas for education to make decisions about life choices in a conscious, informed manner that empowers the person to maintain her/his uniqueness and independence.													
5.4.3 offer self-assessment tools, word associations, storytelling, dreams, journals as appropriate.													
5.4.4 use skills of cultural competence and communicate acceptance of the person's values, beliefs, culture, religion, and socioeconomic background.													

	Where I Want to Be Date:									Check off where you have improved			
	I Knowledge				II Frequency of Activity					III Progress Report			
	Not important	Slightly important	Important	Very important	Do not perform	Less than 1 per week	1–5 per week	6–10 per week	Greater than 10 per week	3 Months	6 Months	9 Months	12 Months
5.4.5 assist the person in recognizing at-risk patterns/problems/needs for potential or existing health situations (e.g., personal habits, personal and family health history, age-related risk factors), and also assist in recognizing opportunities to enhance well-being.													
5.4.6 engage the person in problem-solving dialogue in relation to living with changes secondary to illness and treatment.													
5.5 Implementation: Each person's plan of holistic care is prioritized and holistic nursing interventions are implemented accordingly.													
Standards of Practice Holistic nurses: 5.5.1 implement the mutually created plan of care within the context of assisting the person toward the higher potential of health and well-being.													
5.5.2 support and promote the person's capacity for the highest level of participation and problem solving in the plan of care and collaborate with other health team members when appropriate.													
5.5.3 use holistic nursing skills in implementing care including cultural competency and all ways of knowing.													
5.5.4 advocate that the person's plan, choices, and unique healing journey be honored.													
5.5.5 provide care that is clear about and respectful of the economic parameters of practice, balancing justice with compassion.													

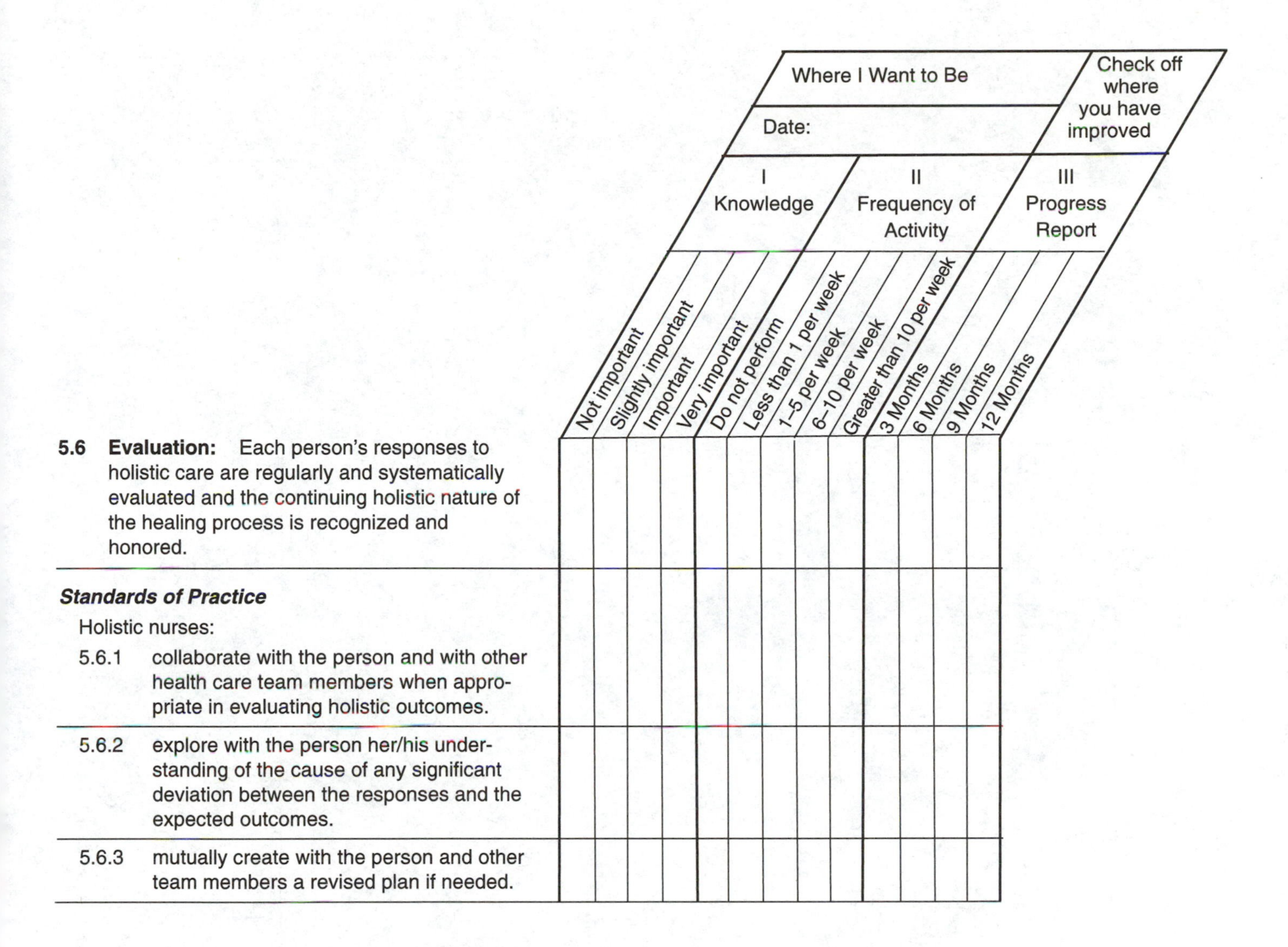

	Where I Want to Be									Check off where you have improved			
	Date:												
	I Knowledge				II Frequency of Activity					III Progress Report			
	Not important	Slightly important	Important	Very important	Do not perform	Less than 1 per week	1–5 per week	6–10 per week	Greater than 10 per week	3 Months	6 Months	9 Months	12 Months
5.6 Evaluation: Each person's responses to holistic care are regularly and systematically evaluated and the continuing holistic nature of the healing process is recognized and honored.													
Standards of Practice Holistic nurses: 5.6.1 collaborate with the person and with other health care team members when appropriate in evaluating holistic outcomes.													
5.6.2 explore with the person her/his understanding of the cause of any significant deviation between the responses and the expected outcomes.													
5.6.3 mutually create with the person and other team members a revised plan if needed.													

APPENDIX B

AHNA HOLISTIC NURSING CORE VALUES AUDIT

INSTRUCTIONS

KEY: Recognition (R): awareness of the 5 AHNA Core Values
Integration (I): application of the 5 AHNA Core Values

Complete the following AHNA Holistic Nursing Core Values Audit, which helps you recognize the consistency of what you value with the values of your boss/manager and the hospital/clinic/corporation.

Step 1: Review the 5 AHNA Core Values and component parts.
Step 2: In the first column (Personal) place an **R** (Recognition) and an **I** (Integration) for all components of the 5 Core Values that apply to you.
Step 3: In the second column (Boss/Manager) place an **R** (Recognition) and an **I** (Integration) for all components of the 5 Core Values that apply to your boss/manager.
Step 4: In the third column (Hospital/Clinic/Corporation) place an **R** (Recognition) and an **I** (Integration) for all components of the 5 Core Values that apply to your hospital/clinic/corporation.
Step 5: Add all the **R**s and **I**s for each of the six columns for a total score. The total possible score for each column is 15.

HOW TO USE THE SCORES

Step 1: Personal Core Values Audit

A. How different are the Rs and Is in your personal audit? (You will probably find a higher score in the **R** column than in the **I** column)
B. Which core values that you already recognized would you like to integrate in your practice?
C. What can you do on a daily basis to increase your recognition and integration of all components of the 5 AHNA Core Values?
D. Can you find a partner or mentor (or be a mentor to a colleague) to help you achieve your goals in recognizing and integrating the 5 AHNA Core Values?

Step 2: Boss/Manager Core Values Audit

- **A.** How different are the Rs and Is in your boss/manager audit?
- **B.** Which core values would you like your boss/manager to recognize and integrate in the workplace?
- **C.** How different are the Rs and the Is in your personal audit compared to those in your boss/manager audit?
- **D.** Who might partner or mentor your boss/manager to better recognize and integrate the 5 AHNA Core Values?
- **E.** How can you educate your boss/manager to support the staff in the recognition and integration of the 5 AHNA Core Values?

Step 3: Hospital/Clinic/Corporation Core Values Audit

- **A** How different are the Rs and Is in your hospital/clinic/corporation audit?
- **B.** Which core values would you like your hospital/clinic/corporation to recognize and integrate in the workplace?
- **C.** How different are the Rs and the Is in your personal audit compared to those in your hospital/clinic/corporation audit?
- **D.** How different are the Rs and the Is in your boss/manager audit as compared to the hospital/clinic/corporation?
- **E.** Who might partner or mentor key people in your hospital/clinic/corporation to better recognize and integrate the 5 AHNA Core Values?
- **F.** How can you educate the vice-presidents and CEOs to support the staff in the recognition and integration of the 5 AHNA Core Values?

Step 4: Choices and Decisions

If you are unable to more closely align your personal goals with that of your boss/manager and hospital/clinic/corporation, do you need to consider another practice setting and a more healing environment?

AHNA Holistic Nursing Core Values Audit

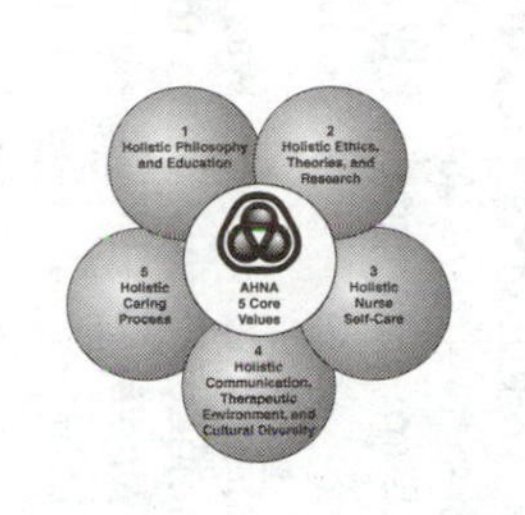

SUMMARY AHNA CORE VALUES

	Personal Recognition and Integration of 5 AHNA Core Values		**Boss/Manager** Recognition and Integration of 5 AHNA Core Values		**Hospital/Clinic/Corporation** Recognition and Integration of 5 AHNA Core Values	
Core Value 1. Holistic Philosophy and Education	R	I	R	I	R	I
1.1 Holistic Philosophy: Holistic nurses develop and expand their conceptual framework and overall philosophy in the art and science of holistic nursing to model, practice, teach, and conduct research in the most effective manner possible.						
1.2 Holistic Education: Holistic nurses acquire and maintain current knowledge and competency in holistic nursing practice.						
Core Value 2. Holistic Ethics, Theories, and Research						
2.1 Holistic Ethics: Holistic nurses hold to a professional ethic of caring and healing that seeks to preserve wholeness and dignity of self, students, colleagues, and the person who is receiving care in all practice settings, be it in health promotion, birthing centers, acute or chronic health care facilities, end-of-life care centers, or in homes.						
2.2 Holistic Nursing Theories: Holistic nurses recognize that holistic nursing theories provide the framework for all aspects of holistic nursing practice and transformational leadership.						
2.3 Holistic Nursing and Related Research: Holistic nurses provide care and guidance to persons through nursing interventions and holistic therapies consistent with research findings and other sound evidence.						
Core Value 3. Holistic Nurse Self-Care						
3.1 Holistic Nurse Self-Care: Holistic nurses engage in self-care and further develop their own personal awareness of being an instrument to better serve self and others.						
Core Value 4. Holistic Communication, Therapeutic Environment, and Cultural Diversity						
4.1 Holistic Communication: Holistic nurses engage in holistic communication to ensure that each person experiences the presence of the nurse as authentic and sincere; there is an atmosphere of shared humanness that includes a sense of connectedness and attention reflecting the individual's uniqueness.						
4.2 Therapeutic Environment: Holistic nurses recognize that each person's environment includes everything that surrounds the individual, both the external and the internal (physical, mental, social, emotional, and spiritual) as well as patterns not yet understood.						
4.3 Cultural Diversity: Holistic nurses recognize each person as a whole body-mind-spirit being and mutually create a plan of care consistent with cultural background, health beliefs, sexual orientation, values, and preferences.						
Core Value 5. Holistic Caring Process						
5.1 Assessment: Each person is assessed holistically using appropriate traditional and holistic methods while the uniqueness of the person is honored.						
5.2 Patterns/Problems/Needs: Actual and potential patterns/problems/needs and life processes related to health, wellness, disease, or illness which may or may not facilitate well-being are identified and prioritized.						
5.3 Outcomes: Each person's actual or potential patterns/problems/needs have appropriate outcomes specified.						
5.4 Therapeutic Care Plan: Each person engages with the holistic nurse to mutually create an appropriate plan of care that focuses on health promotion, recovery or restoration, or peaceful dying so that the person is as independent as possible.						
5.5 Implementation: Each person's plan of holistic care is prioritized and holistic nursing interventions are implemented accordingly.						
5.6 Evaluation: Each person's responses to holistic care are regularly and systematically evaluated and the continuing holistic nature of the healing process is recognized and honored.						
Total Possible Score for Each Column—15	15	15	15	15	15	15
Actual Score for Each Column						

Sample Filled Out Form: Initial AHNA Core Values Audit

SUMMARY AHNA CORE VALUES	Personal Recognition and Integration of 5 AHNA Core Values		Boss/Manager Recognition and Integration of 5 AHNA Core Values		Hospital/Clinic/Corporation Recognition and Integration of 5 AHNA Core Values	
Core Value 1. Holistic Philosophy and Education	R	I	R	I	R	I
1.1 Holistic Philosophy: Holistic nurses develop and expand their conceptual framework and overall philosophy in the art and science of holistic nursing to model, practice, teach, and conduct research in the most effective manner possible.	R	I	R		R	
1.2 Holistic Education: Holistic nurses acquire and maintain current knowledge and competency in holistic nursing practice.	R	I				
Core Value 2. Holistic Ethics, Theories, and Research						
2.1 Holistic Ethics: Holistic nurses hold to a professional ethic of caring and healing that seeks to preserve wholeness and dignity of self, students, colleagues, and the person who is receiving care in all practice settings, be it in health promotion, birthing centers, acute or chronic health care facilities, end-of-life care centers, or in homes.	R	I	R			
2.2 Holistic Nursing Theories: Holistic nurses recognize that holistic nursing theories provide the framework for all aspects of holistic nursing practice and transformational leadership.	R	I				
2.3 Holistic Nursing and Related Research: Holistic nurses provide care and guidance to persons through nursing interventions and holistic therapies consistent with research findings and other sound evidence.	R	I				
Core Value 3. Holistic Nurse Self-Care						
3.1 Holistic Nurse Self-Care: Holistic nurses engage in self-care and further develop their own personal awareness of being an instrument to better serve self and others.	R	I				
Core Value 4. Holistic Communication, Therapeutic Environment, and Cultural Diversity						
4.1 Holistic Communication: Holistic nurses engage in holistic communication to ensure that each person experiences the presence of the nurse as authentic and sincere; there is an atmosphere of shared humanness that includes a sense of connectedness and attention reflecting the individual's uniqueness.	R	I	R		R	
4.2 Therapeutic Environment: Holistic nurses recognize that each person's environment includes everything that surrounds the individual, both the external and the internal (physical, mental, social, emotional, and spiritual) as well as patterns not yet understood.	R	I				
4.3 Cultural Diversity: Holistic nurses recognize each person as a whole body-mind-spirit being and mutually create a plan of care consistent with cultural background, health beliefs, sexual orientation, values, and preferences.	R	I				
Core Value 5. Holistic Caring Process						
5.1 Assessment: Each person is assessed holistically using appropriate traditional and holistic methods while the uniqueness of the person is honored.	R	I	R			
5.2 Patterns/Problems/Needs: Actual and potential patterns/problems/needs and life processes related to health, wellness, disease, or illness which may or may not facilitate well-being are identified and prioritized.	R	I	R			
5.3 Outcomes: Each person's actual or potential patterns/problems/needs have appropriate outcomes specified.	R	I	R			
5.4 Therapeutic Care Plan: Each person engages with the holistic nurse to mutually create an appropriate plan of care that focuses on health promotion, recovery or restoration, or peaceful dying so that the person is as independent as possible.	R	I	R			
5.5 Implementation: Each person's plan of holistic care is prioritized and holistic nursing interventions are implemented accordingly.	R	I	R			
5.6 Evaluation: Each person's responses to holistic care are regularly and systematically evaluated and the continuing holistic nature of the healing process is recognized and honored.	R	I	R			
Total Possible Score for Each Column—15	15	15	15	15	15	15
Actual Score for Each Column	15	15	9	0	2	0

This AHNA Holistic Nursing Core Values Audit in this example illustrates that the holistic nurse clearly recognizes and integrates the 5 AHNA core values. The Boss/Manager and the Hospital/Clinic/Corporation recognize only a few aspects with no integration of the 5 AHNA core values. The question that this nurse asked herself was if the differences and disparities between the personal and the boss/manager and the hospital/clinic/corporation remained this far apart, did she have a need for a more compatible practice setting.

She elected to stay in her practice setting as a nurse educator. She asked five holistic nurses within the 300-bed hospital to work with her to provide a one-day workshop for the staff to increase awareness of aspects of the 5 AHNA Core Values. They also designed a one-year plan with specific goals at three-month intervals.

A one-day workshop on holistic nursing and self-care was designed and approved. The course included information from the *AHNA Core Curriculum for Holistic Nursing*. CEUs were given. All nurses went through the course in three months and stated interest in further workshops.

During the next three-month period, brown bag lunches were held on a weekly basis that presented caring-healing interventions included within the *AHNA Core Curriculum*. Various staff members served on the policy and procedures committees to provide guidelines and draft protocols for better integration of holistic nursing and caring-healing interventions into clinical practice.

The next six months involved more in-depth workshops in holistic nursing and caring-healing interventions from the *AHNA Core Curriculum*. Guest speakers and practitioners presented various holistic interventions on a monthly basis. Three nurses were responsible for meeting with nurse managers, upper management, and administration to educate them on holistic nursing, holistic nursing interventions, and strategies to increase the recognition and integration of holistic nursing and the AHNA Core Values.

At the end of the first year 11 staff nurses successfully completed the American Holistic Nurses' Certification Corporation examination process. An ongoing continuing education program in holistic nursing and caring-healing interventions was established. A one-year repeat AHNA Core Values Audit indicated a greater consistency between a majority of nurses' personal core values with that of the boss/managers and hospital/clinic/corporation.

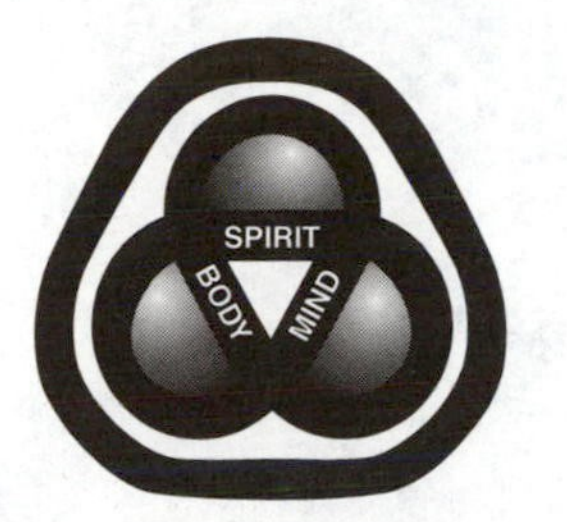

APPENDIX C

THE AHNA CERTIFICATE ENDORSEMENT PROGRAM

Aromatherapy for Health Professionals
R.J. Buckle Associates, LLC
P.O. Box 868
Hunter, NY 12442
(518) 263-4402
Home Page: *www.RJBUCKLE@DELPHI.com*

Healing Touch Program
Colorado Center for Healing Touch
198 Union Blvd., #214
Lakewood, CO 80228
(303) 989-0581
E-mail: *ccheal@aol.com*
Home Page: *www.healingtouch.com*

Nurses Certificate Program in Interactive Imagery℠
Beyond Ordinary Nursing
P.O. Box 8177
Foster City, CA 94404
(650) 570-6157
E-mail: *ncpII@aol.com*
Home Page: *http://members.aol.com/NCPII/NCPII.html*

Nurses Certificate Program in AMMA Therapy®
The New Center College
6801 Jericho Turnpike, Suite 300
Syosset, NY 11791-4413
(800) 922-7337
Home Page: *www.newcenter.edu/certprogram.htm*

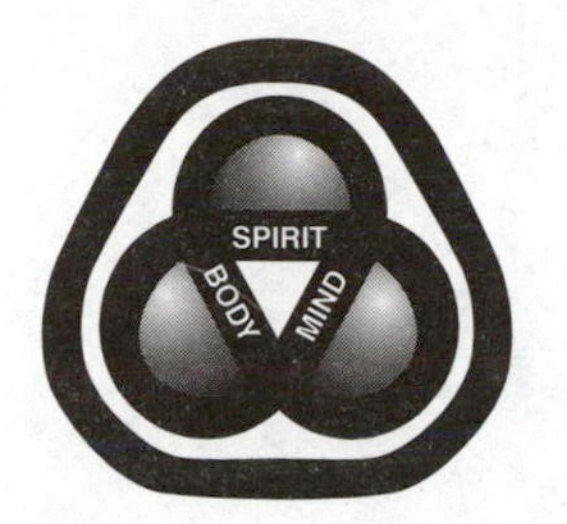

APPENDIX D

GRADUATE NURSING PROGRAMS IN THE UNITED STATES WITH A SPECIALTY IN HOLISTIC NURSING

While many nursing graduate programs in the United States are based on holistic philosophy and guided by a holistic nursing theory, there are five programs offering a Master's degree with opportunity to focus in the practice:

Beth El College of Nursing and Health Care
University of Colorado, Colorado Springs
Master of Science in Nursing with a minor in Holistic Health Nursing

College of New Rochelle
School of Nursing
New Rochelle, NY
Master of Science Program, Clinical Specialist in Holistic Nursing

Flordia Atlantic University
College of Nursing
Boca Raton, FL
Master of Science in Nursing with an Integrative Approach to Holistic Nursing track

New York University
School of Education, Division of Nursing
New York, NY
Master's Degree Program, Advanced Practice Nursing: Holistic Nursing

Tennessee State University
School of Nursing
Nashville, TN
MSN Degree in Holistic Nursing

Also, at the time of this writing, there are several Nurse Practitioner Programs and Clinical Nurse Specialist Programs offering tracks or specialities in Integrative and Complementary Modalities.

APPENDIX E

APPLICATION OF AHNA STANDARDS OF PRACTICE WITH IMAGERY INTERVENTIONS

INTRODUCTION

The following guidelines are presented as an example of how the **AHNA Standards of Holistic Nursing Practice** can serve as a model for integration of a holistic modality such as imagery interventions which are frequently incorporated into clinical practice, education, research, and holistic nurse self-care. These guidelines illustrate the integrations of the modality of imagery with the five Core Values of the Standards.

A general description of imagery is that it is an interface between body, mind, and spirit. It assists a person in the conscious expression from the depths of their inner experience. Imagery is a strategy for evoking change in body, attitudes, behaviors, and beliefs. It is also a method of achieving the fullest potential of casting inner information and action into the present moment or future state for high-level wellness or peaceful dying. The following definitions listed are those most frequently used in imagery interventions:

Body-Mind Imagery: the conscious formation of an image that is directed to a body area or activity that requires attention or increased energy.
Clinical Imagery: the conscious formation of the power of the imagination with the intention of activating biologic, psychologic, or spiritual healing.
Correct Biologic Imagery: biologically accurate images that are visualized to send messages to physiologic processes.
End-State Imagery: images that contain specified imagined hopes and goals (e.g., wound healing).
Guided Imagery: a highly structured imagery technique where a holistic nurse guides a person to bring to mind an image of something and then directly interact with this image, often in dialogue.
Imagery Process: internal experiences of memories, dreams, fantasies, and visions, sometimes involving one, several, or more of the senses, serving as a bridge for connecting a person's body-mind-spirit.
Imagery Rehearsal: an imagery technique designed to rehearse behaviors or prepare for activities or procedures.
Impromptu Imagery: the nurse's introduction of his or her spontaneous, intuitive images or perceptions into the therapeutic intervention.
Package Imagery: commercial tapes that have general images.
Relationship Imagery: imagery technique designed to explore relationships.
Spontaneous Imagery: the unexpected reception of an image, as if it "bubbled up," entering the stream of consciousness.
Standards of Practice: a group of statements describing the expected level of care by a holistic nurse.

Symbolic Imagery: inner images that represent a person's deeper knowledge. Occurring in the form of metaphors or symbols, they may be immediately translatable to rational verbal thought, or their meaning may slowly emerge over time.
Transpersonal Imagery: images that connect one to expanded (i.e., beyond personality) levels of consciousness, such as imagining one's body as a mountain and beginning to feel an inner quality of immovable strength and solidity.
Visualization: the use of external images (e.g., religious painting, written word, nature photograph) to evoke internal imagery experiences that energize desired emotions, qualities, outcomes, and goals.

IMAGERY INTERVENTIONS INTEGRATING THE AHNA STANDARDS OF NURSING PRACTICE

Core Value 1. Holistic Philosophy and Education
Core Value 2. Holistic Ethics, Theories, and Research
Core Value 3. Holistic Nurse Self-Care
Core Value 4. Holistic Communication, Therapeutic Environment, and Cultural Diversity
Core Value 5. Holistic Caring Process

GUIDELINES

The Guidelines for Imagery Interventions:

- are used in conjunction with the American Nurses' Association Standards of Practice, the state nurses practice acts, the AHNA Standards of Holistic Nursing Practice, and the specific specialty standards where holistic nurses practice.
- contain five core values that are followed by a description and Standards of Practice action statements. Depending on the setting or area of practice, holistic nurses may or may not use all of these action statements.
- draw on modalities derived from a number of explanatory models, of which biomedicine is only one model.
- reflect the diverse nursing activities in which holistic nurses are engaged.
- serve holistic nurses in personal life, clinical and private practice, education, research, and community service.

CORE VALUE 1. HOLISTIC PHILOSOPHY AND EDUCATION

1.1 Holistic Philosophy

Holistic nurses develop and expand their conceptual framework and overall philosophy with imagery interventions and integrate the art and science of holistic nursing to model, practice, teach, and conduct research in the most effective manner possible.

Standards of Practice

Holistic nurses:

1.1.1 recognize the person's capacity for self-healing and the importance of supporting the natural development and unfolding of that capacity when using imagery interventions.

1.1.2 support, share, and recognize expertise and competency in imagery interventions and in holistic nursing practice that is used in many diverse clinical and community settings.

1.1.3 participate in person-centered care by using imagery interventions and serve as a partner, coach, and mentor who actively listens and supports others in reaching personal goals.
1.1.4 focus on imagery interventions and strategies to bring harmony, unity, and healing to the nursing profession.
1.1.5 communicate with traditional health care practitioners about appropriate imagery intervention referrals to other holistic practitioners when needed.
1.1.6 interact with professional organizations in a leadership or membership capacity at local, state, national, and international levels to further expand the knowledge and practice of holistic nursing, imagery interventions, and awareness of holistic health issues.

1.2 Holistic Education

Holistic nurses acquire and maintain current knowledge and competency in imagery interventions and holistic nursing practice.

Standards of Practice

Holistic nurses:
1.2.1 participate in activities of continuing education in imagery interventions and related fields that have relevance to holistic nursing practice.
1.2.2 identify areas of knowledge with imagery interventions from nursing and various fields such as biomedicine, epidemiology, behavioral medicine, cultural and social theories.
1.2.3 continually develop and standardize imagery interventions and holistic nursing guidelines, protocols and practice to promote competency in holistic nursing practice and assure quality of care to individuals.
1.2.4 use the results of quality care activities with imagery interventions to initiate change in holistic nursing practice.
1.2.5 may seek certification in imagery interventions and holistic nursing as one means of advancing the philosophy and practice of holistic nursing.

CORE VALUE 2. HOLISTIC ETHICS, THEORIES, AND RESEARCH

2.1 Holistic Ethics

Holistic nurses use imagery interventions and hold to a professional ethic of caring and healing that seeks to preserve wholeness and dignity of self, students, colleagues, and the person who is receiving care in all practice settings, be it in health promotion, birthing centers, acute or chronic care facilities, end-of-life centers, or homes.

Standards of Practice

Holistic nurses:
2.1.1 identify the ethics of caring and its contribution to unity of self, others, nature, and God/Life Force/Absolute/Transcendent as central to holistic nursing practice when using imagery interventions.
2.1.2 integrate standards of holistic nursing practice and guidelines for imagery interventions with applicable state laws and regulations governing nursing practice.
2.1.3 engage in imagery interventions and activities that respect, nurture, and enhance the integral relationship with the earth, and advocate for the well-being of the global community's economy, education, and social justice.

2.1.4 advocate for the rights of patients to have educated choices into their plan of care when imagery interventions are used.
2.1.5 participate in peer evaluation to ensure knowledge and competency in holistic nursing practice and imagery interventions.
2.1.6 protect the personal privacy and confidentiality of individuals, especially with health care agencies and managed care organizations, when using imagery interventions.

2.2 Holistic Theories

Holistic nurses recognize that holistic nursing theories provide the framework for use of all aspects of holistic nursing practice, imagery interventions, and transformational leadership.

Standards of Practice

Holistic nurses:
2.2.1 strive to use nursing theories and imagery interventions theories to develop holistic nursing practice and transformational leadership.
2.2.2 interpret, use, and document imagery interventions information relevant to a person's care according to a theoretical framework.

2.3 Holistic Nursing and Related Research

Holistic nurses provide care and guidance to persons through nursing interventions and holistic therapies such as imagery interventions consistent with research findings and other sound evidence.

Standards of Practice

Holistic nurses:
2.3.1 use available imagery interventions research and evidence from different explanatory models to mutually create a plan of care with a person.
2.3.2 use expert clinical judgment to select appropriate imagery interventions.
2.3.3 discuss holistic application to clinical situations where rigorous imagery interventions research has not been done.
2.3.4 create an environment conducive to systematic inquiry into healing and health issues by engaging in imagery interventions research or supporting and utilizing the research of others.
2.3.5 disseminate imagery interventions research findings at meetings and through publications to further develop the foundation and practice of holistic nursing.
2.3.6 provide consultation services on holistic nursing interventions such as imagery interventions to persons and communities based on research.

CORE VALUE 3. HOLISTIC NURSE SELF-CARE

Holistic Nurse Self-Care

Holistic nurses engage in self-care and further develop their own personal awareness of being an instrument of healing to better serve self and others by using imagery interventions.

Standards of Practice

Holistic nurses:

3.1.1 recognize that a person's body-mind-spirit has healing capacities that can be enhanced and supported through imagery interventions and self-care practices.

3.1.2 identify and integrate imagery interventions and self-care strategies to enhance their physical, psychological, sociological, and spiritual well-being.

3.1.3 recognize and address at-risk health patterns and begin the process of change by using imagery interventions.

3.1.4 consciously cultivate awareness and understanding about the deeper meaning, purpose, inner strengths, and connections with self, others, nature, and God/Life Force/Absolute/Transcendent with the use of imagery interventions.

3.1.5 use imagery interventions and a clear intention to care for self and to seek a sense of balance, harmony, and joy in daily life.

3.1.6 participate in the evolutionary imagery and holistic process with the understanding that crisis creates opportunity in any setting.

CORE VALUE 4. HOLISTIC COMMUNICATION, THERAPEUTIC ENVIRONMENT, AND CULTURAL DIVERSITY

Holistic Communication

Holistic nurses use imagery interventions to engage in holistic communication to ensure that each person experiences the presence of the nurse as authentic and sincere; there is an atmosphere of shared humanness that includes a sense of connectedness and attention reflecting the individual's uniqueness.

Standards of Practice

Holistic nurses:

4.1.1 develop an awareness of the most frequently encountered challenges to holistic communication to integrate imagery interventions.

4.1.2 increase therapeutic and cultural competence skills to enhance their effectiveness through listening to themselves and others when integrating imagery interventions.

4.1.3 explore with each person those imagery interventions and strategies that can assist her/him, as desired, to understand the deeper meaning, purpose, inner strengths, and connections with self, others, nature, and God/Life Force/Absolute/Transcendent.

4.1.4 recognize that imagery interventions can enhance holistic communication and awareness of individuals is a continuously evolving multi-level exchange that offers itself through dreams, images, symbols, sensations, meditations, and prayers.

4.1.5 respect the person's health trajectory, which may be incongruent with conventional wisdom when using imagery interventions.

Therapeutic Environment

Holistic nurses recognize that each person's environment includes everything that surrounds the individual, both the external and internal (physical, mental, emotional, social, and spiritual), as well as patterns not yet understood when using imagery interventions.

Standards of Practice

Holistic nurses:

4.2.1 promote environments conducive to experiencing healing, wholeness, and harmony, and care for the person in as healthy an environment as possible when using imagery interventions.

4.2.2 work toward creating organizations that value sacred space and environments that enhance healing when using imagery interventions.

4.2.3 integrate holistic principles, standards, policies, and procedures in relation to environmental safety and emergency preparedness when using imagery interventions.

4.2.4 recognize that the well-being of the ecosystem of the planet is a prior determining condition for the well-being of the human when using imagery interventions.

4.2.5 promote social networks and social environments where healing can take place when using imagery interventions.

4.3 Cultural Diversity

Holistic nurses recognize each person as a whole being of body-mind-spirit and mutually create a plan of care consistent with cultural backgrounds, health beliefs, sexual orientation, values, and preferences when using imagery interventions.

Standards of Practice

Holistic nurses:

4.3.1 assess and incorporate the person's cultural practices, values, beliefs, meaning of health, illness, and risk behaviors in care and health education when using imagery interventions.

4.3.2 use appropriate community resources and experts to extend their understanding of different cultures when using imagery interventions.

4.3.3 assess for discriminatory practices and change as necessary when using imagery interventions.

4.3.4 identify discriminatory health care practices as they impact the person and engage in effective nondiscriminatory practices when using imagery interventions.

CORE VALUE 5. HOLISTIC CARING PROCESS

5.1 Assessment

Each person is assessed holistically using appropriate traditional and holistic methods such as imagery interventions while the uniqueness of the person is honored.

Standards of Practice

Holistic nurses:

5.1.1 use an assessment process including appropriate traditional and holistic methods such as imagery interventions to systematically gather information.

5.1.2 value all types of knowing including intuition when gathering data from a person and validate this intuitive knowledge with the person when appropriate prior to imagery interventions.

5.2 Patterns/Problems/Needs

Each person's actual and potential patterns/problems/needs and life processes related to health, wellness, disease, or illness that may or may not facilitate well-being are identified and prioritized when using imagery interventions.

Standards of Practice

Holistic nurses:

5.2.1 assist the person to access inner wisdom that can provide opportunities to enhance and support growth, development, and movement toward health and well-being when using imagery interventions.

5.2.2 collect data and collaborate with the person and health care team members as appropriate to identify and record a list of actual and potential patterns/problems/needs when using imagery interventions.

5.2.3 use collected data to formulate an etiology of the person's identified actual or potential patterns/problems/needs when using imagery interventions.

5.2.4 make referrals to other holistic practitioners or traditional therapist when appropriate for imagery interventions.

5.3 Outcomes

Each person's actual or potential patterns/problems/needs have appropriate outcomes specified when using imagery interventions.

Standards of Practice

Holistic nurses:

5.3.1 honor the person in all phases of her/his healing process regardless of expectations or outcomes when using imagery interventions.

5.3.2 identify and partner with the person to specify measurable outcomes and realistic goals when using imagery interventions.

5.4 Therapeutic Care Plan

Each person engages with the holistic nurse to mutually create an appropriate plan of care that focuses on health promotion, recovery, restoration, or peaceful dying so that the person is as independent as possible when using imagery interventions.

Standards of Practice

Holistic nurses:

5.4.1 partner with the person in a mutual decision process to create a health care plan for each pattern/problem/need or opportunity to enhance health and well-being when using imagery interventions.

5.4.2 help a person identify areas for education to make decisions about life choices in a conscious, informed manner that empowers the person to maintain her/his uniqueness and independence when using imagery interventions.

5.4.3 offer self-assessment tools, word associations, storytelling, dreams, journals as appropriate when using imagery interventions.

5.4.4 use skills of cultural competence and communicate acceptance of the person's values, beliefs, culture, religion, and socioeconomic background when using imagery interventions.
5.4.5 assist the person in recognizing at-risk patterns/problems/needs for potential or existing health situations (e.g., personal habits, personal and family health history, age-related risk factors), and also assist in recognizing opportunities to enhance well-being when using imagery interventions.
5.4.6 engage the person in problem-solving dialogue in relation to living with changes secondary to illness and treatment when using imagery interventions.

5.5 Implementation

Each person's plan of holistic care is prioritized and holistic nursing interventions are implemented accordingly when using imagery interventions.

Standards of Practice

Holistic nurses:
5.5.1 implement the mutually created plan of care within the context of assisting the person toward the higher potential of health and well-being when using imagery interventions.
5.5.2 support and promote the person's capacity for the highest level of participation and problem solving in the plan of care and collaborate with other health team members when appropriate when using imagery interventions.
5.5.3 use holistic nursing skills in implementing care including cultural competency and all ways of knowing when using imagery interventions.
5.5.4 advocate that the person's plan, choices, and unique healing journey be honored when using imagery interventions.
5.5.5 provide care that is clear about and respectful of the economic parameters of practice, balancing justice with compassion, when using imagery interventions.

5.6 Evaluation

Each person's responses to holistic care are regularly and systematically evaluated and the continuing holistic nature of the healing process is recognized and honored when using imagery interventions.

Standards of Practice

Holistic nurses:
5.6.1 collaborate with the person and with other health care team members when appropriate in evaluating holistic outcomes when using imagery interventions.
5.6.2 explore with the person her/his understanding of the cause of any significant deviation between the responses and the expected outcomes when using imagery interventions.
5.6.3 mutually create with the person and other team members a revised plan if needed when using imagery interventions.

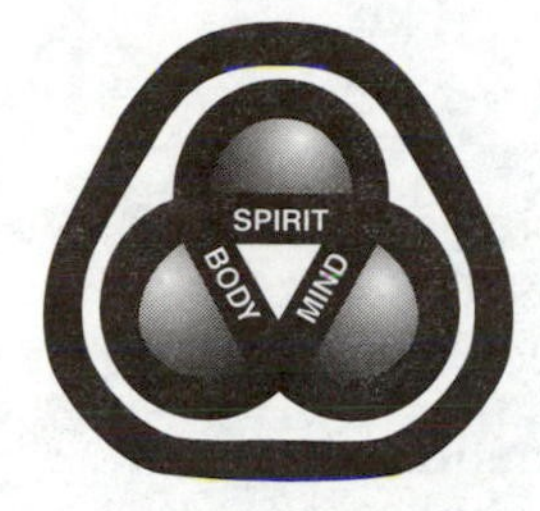

Index